T0067363

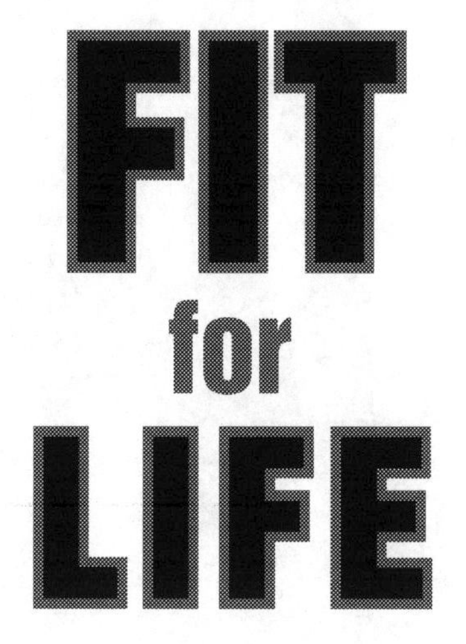

It's Never Too Late to BE HEALTHY

Wyndy C. Buckner

Edited by Jeanette Morris

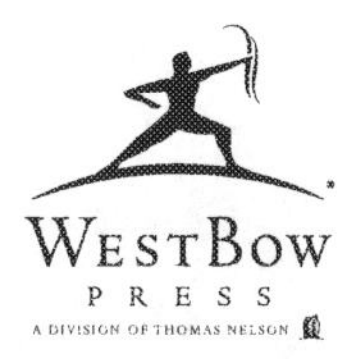

Consulting expert: Connie Simmons, M.Ed., Fit for Life Educator
Consulting expert: Major Gregory Simmons, B.S.

WestBow Press books may be ordered through booksellers or by contacting:

WestBow Press
A Division of Thomas Nelson
1663 Liberty Drive
Bloomington, IN 47403
www.westbowpress.com
1-(866) 928-1240

ISBN: 978-1-4497-1528-1 (sc)
ISBN: 978-1-4497-1527-4 (e)

Library of Congress Control Number: 2011926312

Printed in the United States of America

WestBow Press rev. date: 4/20/2011

Contents

Acknowledgments

Special thanks to those who labored together with me on this book.

To my husband, Mike, who spent as many hours transferring my handwritten pages into the computer as I did writing them out longhand. For his patience in fixing, editing, organizing, and helping me develop this workbook for you, my students.

To my daughter, Connie. Words are not enough to express my gratitude for all of your support, ideas, and for all the time you spent patiently listening. For your encouragement to press forward in the difficult times I had when I started exercising. I treasure our times working out together at the YMCA. Your coaching, your presence, and your confidence in me have sustained me more than you will ever know. I love you.

To Michael, who was one of the first to taste-test my new lifestyle. I had to learn how to cook in a completely new way. Michael was very kind in letting me know if something was edible (or not).

To my sister, Viv, who started me on this journey by placing a book in my hands. God used this book to completely change the direction of my life—a life that was held captive by Satan through an unhealthy lifestyle—to a healthy one that was transformed by God and His Holy Word.

To Jeanette, my God-sent editor. Thank you for all of your work, patience, and time. Your expertise in helping me develop *Fit for Life* into a workbook is invaluable. I love using quotes, and so I say, "I couldn't have done it without you" (from *Balto*, one of my favorite movies). You are one of those whom God placed on my journey's path. Only He knew which roads we each needed to travel in order to arrive at stop signs on the same crossroads at the same time! We serve an awesome God.

To Steve, for all of your work in helping me create this workbook. I believe God chooses people's paths in life for special reasons. You passed through my life just when I needed it. We serve an awesome God, and I thank Him for choosing you to be one of my God-sent editors.

Most of all, I give God the glory, and I thank Him for giving me the revelation that led to Wyndy's Story. Because of His love and saving grace, I have found total freedom in all areas of my life.

Introduction

Every ridiculous diet one can imagine already seems to exist. Everywhere we look, somebody has found "the cure." Store shelves are filling with diet pills, powders, and packaged meals. Specialists promote surgery, exercise programs, and therapies of all kinds. The list goes on and on. Nevertheless, the fact remains that a worldwide epidemic of unhealthy living has caused a dangerous and even deadly way of life for millions of people.

There is a concern in every field of expertise that something needs to be done to stop this epidemic. It's time we Christians wake up and recognize this unhealthy lifestyle for what it is: *sin!* As believers, we need to embrace the total truth in God's Word. He instructs us to care for our physical body as well as our spiritual body. This can be done.

Throughout this course, we will discuss and explore how God, in His awesome wisdom, designed our bodies to function in a physical sense. I am not a medical doctor, nor am I giving you, the student, *any* medical advice. I am, however, going to show you a different approach to the epidemic in which our culture is "trapped" today. My reference book will be God's Word, the Holy Bible. Bear in mind that God is calling me to teach you how to care for your body physically; pastors are primarily called to nurture your spiritual life. Two different kinds of teachers, but both teaching from the same Book.

The lessons in *Fit for Life* come in four sections. Section one, "The Trap," demonstrates the trap that captures us. Section two, "The Plague," reveals Satan's purpose behind stealing our physical health. Section three, "The Dwelling," stresses biblical virtues and teachings necessary for unlocking the traps Satan sets to keep us unhealthy. Section four, "Freedom from Sin's Grasp," presents us with the charge that as believers, we are equipped by God and responsible to Him for making a difference. Changing our lifestyle is not only possible; it can eventually become easy and natural.

My purpose is to show you how to address, recognize, and win this battle. The Trap, The Plague, and The Dwelling offer a powerful revelation designed for you as a believer to expose Satan's traps and deception in creating the largest epidemic known to our culture: an unhealthy lifestyle!

I am not suggesting that food is evil, but that being unhealthy is. Satan has set a trap, and we, as the Church, have fallen into it.

I tried to remove, replace, candy-coat, somehow not use the word "sin" in this book, but the reality is, that's the word the Bible uses! We've been educated about, preached to about, prayed for about, and repented of this one word. We as Christians are usually okay with the word "sin," but only if we don't have to apply it to ourselves. I replaced it several times when writing this workbook, but God spoke to me, and firmly told me, "No! Keep it in."

I highly recommend journaling your way through this course. As you probably know, journaling entails writing down your thoughts and feelings as you go through life. As you struggle with losing weight and getting your body into shape, it will help to write about each day's journey. You will find some blank pages toward the back of this book that you can use for journaling. Or you may want to buy your own journaling book so you can write up a storm.

Are you ready to be Fit for Life?

Wyndy's Story

How God Changed My Life Forever

Have you ever tried to lose ten pounds? If you are one of the lucky ones who manage to achieve that goal, it's often only a matter of time before those pounds have glued themselves right back on. I have battled obesity most of my life. I had reached the point, and accepted as fact, that I was going to meet the Lord one day while I was still *fat!* I had tried every means of dieting in existence. I knew the steps so well I could have taught a class at the college of dieting. But I couldn't lose those unwanted pounds and keep them off. Why?

In the fall of 2006, my family relocated to Pennsylvania. The following spring, I was at my all-time low—spiritually, physically, emotionally, and socially—and everyday functions seemed to me like climbing Mt. Everest. The black hole into which I was sinking became my new reality. My body hurt all over. My level of depression was at an all-time high. And yes, suicide was an option for me. However, I knew God's Word well enough to know I couldn't follow that path, no matter how I felt.

At my husband's urging, I made an appointment to see a doctor. Next came all the usual tests. Blood work, X-ray of my aching thumb to make sure it was okay (probably just arthritis). My hips hurt too. Some days I could hardly walk, and just lying down was a challenge. I remember how hard it was to hold back my tears as I waited in the examination room. *What's wrong with me? Why do I feel like this?* It was one of the darkest moments of my life. My doctor ordered tests and reassured me that the blood work would show if any problems existed. Nevertheless, I felt completely alone and defeated.

Two weeks later, I sat in the doctor's office again, not feeling any better, but knowing I had taken the right step. I figured my problem had to be physical, you know, middle age—and all of the hurdles that go along with it. The crying, mood swings, aching joints, the night sweats, lack of desire to do anything but stay in my room. I just knew she was going to say old age or mid-life crisis. But she didn't.

The results were back. My *good* cholesterol, HDL, was acceptable. My *bad* cholesterol, LDL, was acceptable as well. Blood pressure good, sugar good, thyroid good, but my C-reactive protein was very high. *My what?*

The doctor explained, "Your C-reactive protein measures levels of inflammation in blood vessels, a marker for many types of diseases. Arthritis could be a concern, especially rheumatoid arthritis. Is there a history of arthritis in your family?"

Yes, on both sides! She ordered additional blood work and had me schedule a follow-up appointment in two weeks.

"God, where are you?" I cried. "I know you can rescue me. I don't understand what's happening." Psalm 91 is my personal Christian 9-1-1. I read and reread it. As I started praying, certain verses began to speak to my spirit. "Those who live in the shelter of the most High will find rest in the shadow of the Almighty. He alone is my refuge, my place of safety; He is my God, and I am trusting Him. For He will rescue you from every trap, and He will protect you from the fatal plague." Verse 9 says, "If you make the Lord your refuge, if you make the Most High your shelter, no evil will conquer you; no plague will come near your dwelling." I kept reading those two verses and wondering how God would rescue me from every trap, and what He meant that no plague would come near my dwelling. I began asking God, "What trap? What plague?" But these questions marked the beginning of my miraculous turning point.

My sister, who is twelve years older than I, has worked very hard at building a relationship between us. Today, that relationship is a bond "only sisters share." So, it was not a surprise when a book on dieting arrived in the mail from her the next day.

"Have you heard about it?" she asked during our weekly phone call. "It's different than all the other books we've read."

I chuckled as I threw it aside. If there was one thing I didn't feel like doing, it was reading another "fat" book. However, that book stared back at me every time I lounged on the couch. (I didn't feel quite as guilty if I spent the day there vs. the bed in my bedroom.) Eventually I picked it up and flipped through it—casually, of course. But the words seemed to make sense. Much more than any other I'd read. And believe me, I had read many.

Two weeks later, I felt a little better. The book was Dr. Oz's *You on a Diet*, and its advice seemed true to me. I brought it along to my next appointment to show my doctor and get her approval. She just smiled.

The blood results were back. She had good news and not-so-good news. I didn't have rheumatoid arthritis, but I had all the symptoms of arterial inflammation. Even though my cholesterol was acceptable, I was at risk for heart disease and a heart attack! She didn't know if there was any blockage to worry about, but she was concerned enough to run a few more tests before we talked about medication. In the meantime, I needed to get serious about losing weight—very serious.

I felt like someone had slapped my face! The sting of her words pierced my inner being. At that moment, God spoke directly to my spirit. He said, "Greater is He that is in you, than he that is in the world. Who set up camp in your dwelling, Wyndy? You say you love me, so why does someone else control you?" I sat there stunned! I had heard my doctor's warning, but God's warning spoke even louder to me.

At that moment, God lifted the blinders from my eyes, and the healing I had been asking for began to flow through me like a rushing river! Wisdom and understanding of the Trap, the Plague, and my Dwelling flooded every living cell of my body. Sitting alone in that exam room, I heard God calling me to change the food I ate and switch to a healthier lifestyle, one that was pleasing to *Him.*

My burden today is for Christians, and, specifically for Christian children and young people. Doctors claim that today in the United States there is an epidemic of obesity in kids and teens caused by a lethal combination of eating too much food, eating unhealthy food, and too much sitting around.

Rebecca Barlow Jordan wrote: "Life is precious. Each delicate feature is a miracle from God, bearing His mark of ownership, stamped with His approval, created in His image—a heavenly original."

Genesis 1:26 says that we were made in Christ's image! My blue eyes were chosen by God just for me. Every hair on my head is counted (see Luke 12:7). He knows everything there is to know about me and you, and He wants us to keep these bodies of ours working smoothly and efficiently for His glory!

—Wyndy C. Buckner

Section 1
The Trap

Lesson 1

Satan's Snares and How to Recognize Them

This may the most important course you ever take. Our nation has a scary epidemic, and it's called "unhealthiness." The symptoms of this epidemic are frequent sickness, obesity, heart attacks, and other physical problems. In addition, something new is happening; researchers are discovering that, by the millions, kids just like you are becoming more out of shape and overweight than they've ever been before.

If you already eat a balanced, healthy diet, exercise to stay in shape, and keep your weight down, then you probably don't need this class. But if you have a hard time in any of these areas, this course can help set you free from what I call "The Trap."

What is "The Trap," you might be asking. Let's first define the word. A trap is anything planned to deceive, or betray. Does this explanation sound like the vocation of anyone we Christians know? As Dana Carvey, in his best Church Lady voice, used to say, "Hmmmm, maybe Satan?"

When I began seeking God for understanding of "The Trap," I was blown away with the craftiness Satan uses in placing these traps for us to fall into.[1]

Look up the following verses. In the space provided, list the various devices Satan uses to entrap us:

2 Timothy 2:24-26 ______________________________

Psalms 69:22 ______________________________

Ecclesiastes 7:26 ______________________________

When we read the Bible, or attend Sunday worship or Bible studies, we typically apply His Word to our spirit or our spiritual life. But what does God's Word say about our physical life or body?

Look up 2 Corinthians 7:1. Write out the verse here:

____

____

The word "defile" appears in this verse. What do you think "defile" means?

____

____

What is the dictionary definition of "defile"?

____

____

When I recognized "The Trap," my whole thought process began to change. I began seeing food and diet in a totally new way. I was so excited! God began giving me a spiritual understanding regarding how our bodies are to function according to His divine design.

Scripture took on a deeper meaning. "The Trap" came alive for me in Scripture. God began showing me the way He wants us to care for our bodies in the physical sense. It didn't surprise me, then, when He took me to the very beginning—the Garden of Eden—where the first bite of sin took place. At that moment of temptation in the Garden of Eden, Satan set the Trap for the fall of humankind, not only spiritually but also physically. Sin was born!

Unhealthiness is SIN, rebellion is SIN, pride is SIN, disobedience is SIN, neglect of your physical body is SIN. I can just see the doubt reflected on your face. But you are going to hear this word throughout the entire book—the word sin—and I make no apologies.

Scripture tells us we are to die daily to what? Sin. What kinds of sin? ____________

Look up James 4:7. This verse tells us if we know what we ought to be doing, and are not doing it, we're doing what? ______________________________

So, if we know being unhealthy is not good for us, and we're not putting forth any sort of effort to keep our body organs, lungs, joints, muscles, skin, etc.) healthy. We are doing what? ____

If you are pigging out and abusing your body, isn't that a form of rebellion against God? You bet it is! Is disobedience a sin? You bet it is! Just because your body completes the minimum tasks called for in a typical day does not mean you are healthy.

Read John 3: 3, 7: Jesus said that unless you are born again you will not enter the Kingdom of God. What do you think being born again has to do with being healthy or unhealthy? ____

Let's see what the Bible actually says. What are the steps to being born again? Scripture is very clear.

Step 1. (Romans 3:23) ______________________________
______________________________(Recognize you are a sinner)

Step 2. (Romans 10:9) ______________________________
______________________________(Confess and repent of your sins)

Step 3. (Romans 5:1) ______________________________
______________________________(Ask Christ for forgiveness)

What was the purpose of Jesus Christ's coming? He was sacrificed for our sins, that is, for our redemption from sin that we may have life and life more abundantly.

The root of the problem of unhealthiness is SIN. The sin is not in the facts we don't eat right, exercise, or do the things we should. Those things are simply the snares, the "Traps." The sin is abusing our bodies, the temple in which God now lives by His Holy Spirit. The solution to the problem is repentance!

Read John 8:3-11, the story of the woman caught in adultery.

Scripture tells us to go and do what? ______________________________

Well, Wyndy, does that mean I will never sin again? Of course not! It means you will repent more and press toward the mark of completion in Christ. That's why Scripture tells us to die to sin—ONE DAY AT A TIME!

(1) Let me clarify—I know Satan is not omnipresent. Only God is everywhere at once, and Satan can only be in one place at any given time. So when, in this course, I say that Satan is saying or doing something in your life, I am referring to him and his myriads of demon spirits that are scattered throughout our planet.

Lesson 2

Satan's Avenues: The World and the Flesh

Satan traps us by using the World and the Flesh. The World is our society—the system that surrounds us every day. It is, in a sense, ruled by Satan, the "Prince of this World," the "Prince of the Power of the Air."

The Flesh is this old sinful body of ours that constantly pushes us to stick out our chin and abuse the good things God has given us. For example, sleep is a good thing, but we abuse it by sloth and laziness. Money is a good thing, but we abuse it with envy and greed. Sex is a great gift, but we abuse it by immoral behavior. Food is a delicious thing, but we abuse it by gorging ourselves or eating junk foods.

Proverbs 23:21 reads, "The drunkard and the glutton shall come to poverty, and drowsiness shall clothe a man with rags." I don't know why the drunkard and glutton are included together in this verse, but it seems like gluttony is considered a pretty serious problem.

Look up "gluttony" in the dictionary and write the definition here:

____

Gluttony is one of Satan's "Traps." He sets us up to get caught in its snare so that we will fail in our efforts to be healthy.

Changing from an unhealthy lifestyle to a healthy one takes time. Satan has been very clever at creating and developing today's unhealthy lifestyle. He wants you to feel hopelessly unable to change. If you neglect to properly care for your physical body in the way God intended for it to function, you become a victim caught in a sort of spider's web. Unless you can somehow free yourself from that web, you will be destroyed. That old Spider will eat you alive! Satan knows that if he can control your body, he can also control your spirit. I personally know when he gets his sticky hands on me, and I get caught, breaking free becomes a major fight. By yourself, you will not escape. You may do okay for a while, but Satan will set other traps and webs to snare you. However, if you begin looking for the Traps, you will be able to recognize them and sidestep them before they can trip you up. And as you are surely aware, this World and our Flesh are besieged by Satan's Traps.

One of the biggest Traps I have to watch for is my love of sweets. I had to literally die to sugar. Does that mean I can't eat it? No, it means I recognize sugar as a Trap in my life. To avoid being caught in its snares, I can't indulge in it. Did I just see the sugar Trap and, like Superman, destroy it with iron strength? Not hardly.

You on a Diet, by Dr. Oz and Dr. Michael Roizen, offers a clear understanding of the medical perspective on dieting. They show us how our body should function from a medical standpoint. God began showing me from Dr. Oz's book how my body processes food and how addicted my body was to sugar.

There is a process I am going to teach you to go through as each Trap in your World and your Flesh is exposed. As warriors of the Lord, it's our responsibility to be on guard and diligently watch for Traps daily. My goal is to teach you to recognize food Traps.

1. I recognized sugar as a Trap.
2. I confessed to God that I had abused my body (my Flesh) with every sweet delight known to man. Not only that, I enjoyed it, but I was trapped in addiction and bondage. Without God's help, I was too weak to give up sugar.
3. I asked God to forgive me of the sin of abusing His temple. I asked for forgiveness in the areas of gluttony, selfishness, and greed. I recognized my lack of self-control and authority to control my eating. I asked God for help and thanked Him for being such a mighty God. I made a vow to do my best to resist these Traps in my World.

Again, here are the steps to removing Satan's Traps.

1. Recognize the Trap (the one that hinders you) as SIN.
2. Confess that SIN to God.
3. Repent and ask for forgiveness.

This is an ongoing process, no different than confessing wrong in our spiritual lives. We must die daily to sin, both spiritually and physically. (See Matthew 10:38-39.)

One of my dearest friends makes a coconut cake that causes my saliva glands to work overtime. I can just think of that cake and turn into a version of a drooling, teething baby. This cake is four layers high. The frosting is a cooked white frosting that stands in cotton-like peaks all over the cake's top. Then, of course, it's covered with soft, sweet, snow-white coconut. My friend always gives me the honor of slicing it, and I always stand for the occasion. Her masterpiece is beautifully displayed on an elegant cake plate. I carefully cut that cake and, of course, I choose the size of my own slice. Oh, then there's all of that frosting on the knife and on the plate left after the slices are served. I can never resist it. I gorge myself on the cake and frosting.

Soon after God's revelation of the Trap, I felt the yearning for my friend's "cake fix." Our families have developed a special friendship and a six-hour trip was planned. My friend asked, "Should I bake a coconut cake?"

I had been sharing with her what God was doing in my life and health. I immediately told her no. I knew I couldn't resist that cake, and I felt I needed to avoid the trap altogether.

God began speaking to my spirit about control, self-discipline, and putting on the armor of God. He was really challenging me in the areas of faith or, better yet, who is in control, and, strangely, I felt as if God was telling me to call my friend and tell her to bake that cake. Not only bake it, but double the frosting!

Once again, that cake was beautifully and elegantly placed on a crystal cake plate. (Note: God may not lead you in this unusual way.) Of course, the honor of slicing "the cake" was given to me. My hands were actually shaking. I realized I was facing my trap square in the face. When it came time to slice my piece I sensed Satan in the spirit taking great joy and pleasure at my discomfort and vulnerability. I was fighting the urge to slice a small serving rather than a great big one. These few seconds seemed like an eternity. All of a sudden, I had one of those moments when God shows up! I heard this quiet inner voice speak to me: *Wyndy, who's holding the knife?*

I am, Lord.

Wyndy, who's making the decision to eat this cake?

I am Lord.

Wyndy, do you want a small slice or a larger one?

Well, Lord, I really want a big piece.

Wyndy, if you want some cake, then you decide you want it. Don't wolf it down because someone else is controlling your desire.

I made an announcement. "I'm not cutting a little piece. I want a big one. Not only that, I want all of the frosting left on the plate." That cake never tasted as good as it did that night.

I remember the freedom I felt. As I sat there in her kitchen, I made the decision to have a second slice. Not because I couldn't resist the temptation, but because I wanted the cake!

God didn't care if I ate the cake or not, but He did care about the attitude in which I ate it. I truly believe I made Satan fighting mad when I told him how much of that cake *I* had deliberately chosen to eat. He had no power over me! By my conscious choice, I took the power away from him.

Now that experience had a cost. It took my system about three days to completely get over the results of indulging in all that sugar. I had to work at getting my body back to processing my food the healthy way. I increased my activity that week to help balance the extra calories I had eaten.

I want you to also know that I haven't eaten coconut cake since, and I have lost the desire or craving for it. Over time, I lost the desire for sweets altogether. Yes, I still have a bite from time to time, but the uncontrollable yearning is no longer there. I still watch for sugar traps, but I know God has given me the ability to recognize them and resist.

Look up the following Scriptures and write them in the space provided.

James 4:7 ____

____

1 John 4:4 ____

____

____

I have to die daily to the sin of gluttony. Gluttony is gorging ourselves on more food and drink than we should consume. I check out everything I eat for Traps. Believe me, they are there. Everywhere! But there is freedom too! And guess what? When you start treating your body the way God tells you to, you will resist those Traps! You will begin to feel better, and your body will respond to what you have chosen to feed it. Don't let Satan feed you anymore! Remember Philippians 4:13: "For I can do everything with the help of Christ who gives me the strength I need; I can do all things through Christ Jesus who strengthens me" (NLT; NKJ).

Personal Prayer: Lord, thank you for every one of my students. Lord, everyone who reads this book was hand chosen by you, just as you chose me to be the one to reveal your truth about Satan's trap to kill, steal, and destroy our health. Lord, give them the same wisdom and knowledge to discern the food traps in their lives. Help them to use good choices in changing their eating habits from unhealthy ones to healthy ones. Lord, I thank you and stand in the gap for all who ask these things using the powerful name of Jesus. Amen.

Your prayer: ____

____

____

____

____

Lesson 3

Satan's Gift: The First Bite of Sin

Do you remember the part of Wyndy's story where I said that God took me to the beginning? Let's go there together now.

Genesis 1:1 says, "In the beginning God created the Heavens and earth." And then a few verse later, we read about God creating humankind. Genesis 1:26-27: "Then God said, "Let us make people *in Our image,* to be like ourselves." So God created people *in His own image*—God patterned them after Himself, male and female He created them" (emphasis mine). Would God have created an unhealthy image of Himself? Of course not. So what happened to this healthy creation?

Genesis 3:1-6, "Now the serpent (Satan) was the shrewdest of all the creatures the Lord God had made. ' Really?' he asked the woman. 'Did God really say you must not eat any of the fruit?' 'Of course we may eat it,' the woman told him. 'It's only the fruit from the tree at the center of the garden that we are not allowed to eat. God says we must not eat it or even touch it, or we will die!' 'You won't die,' hissed the serpent. 'God knows that your eyes will be opened when you eat it. You will become just like God, *knowing* everything, both *good* and *evil*.' The woman was convinced. The fruit looked so fresh and delicious and it would make her so wise. So she ate some of the fruit. She also gave some to her husband, who was with her, and he ate it too" (emphasis mine).

When Eve committed the first sin, what was the first thing she learned?

____

What was the action of her sin? ____________________
Right, she chomped down on and swallowed the forbidden food God had told her not to eat. From what did God want to protect her? ____________________

Satan, very slowly over time, has re-programmed our brain's natural design of processing and digesting our foods. How has he accomplished this? By changing our body chemistry. Really, but how? By tempting us to eat food that God did not design for us.

Satan has created all of the necessary foods that satisfy this chemical change. He has replaced good for evil. Keep in mind, we were created by God, but it is Satan's mission to destroy us. Satan will not provide us with anything that is good for us, including our food!

Now, being the chocoholic that I am, I imagine the piece of fruit that tempted Eve as being the size of a nice juicy peach, or a very large strawberry, hand-dipped in chocolate (the best there is, of course) not twice, but three times! I can visualize how good that luscious fruit must have tasted. And, of course, I would share with my husband as Eve did, because we both enjoy the moment of pleasure eating something tasty brings us.

So how has Satan deceived us? He has built an empire out of the food industry, which has caused an unhealthy diet to become an all-time epidemic. You might be asking, "How has he accomplished this task?" By placing every type of food we could dream of at our fingertips.

- Fast food courts at the mall
- All-you-can-eat buffets
- Fast food chains
- Donut shops and "quick stops"
- "Coffee" shops
- Drive-through "restaurants"

None of the above specializes in healthy foods, right?

In addition, we eat at every possible opportunity:

- Parties
- Sporting events
- Weddings
- Holidays
- Movies
- Picnics
- Family reunions
- While shopping
- Church functions
- When watching TV

What do we eat and how much? Well, here's my list. These are the types of foods I have eaten at the above functions:

- Cake
- Potato salad
- Baked beans
- Hot dogs
- Fried chicken
- Sweets
- Chips 'n dip
- Macaroni salad
- Chocolate cream pie
- Soda

What about you? Write down your favorite fun foods or comfort foods here:

____________________ ____________________

____________________ ____________________

____________________ ____________________

____________________ ____________________

Fried this, creamed that, loaded with calories or sugar and smothered in fat. How many times have you eaten just one tablespoon of potato salad? Or one bite of cake? Or one sip of soda? Our Western culture has evolved around this lifestyle of eating, and it has become as natural as getting up and going to work. People of all shapes and sizes are affected by today's eating habits. You can suffer from obesity, or be as thin as an underweight Q-tip, and still be unhealthy.

Just as Moses and Aaron were sent by God to get in Pharaoh's face, I believe God has spoken to me. This is what the Lord, the God of Israel, said to pharaoh, and what I want to say to Satan: "Let my people go!" God will expose Satan's trap of deception and you, as the believer, will be shown the truth if you make the decision to exercise your God-given free will.

You can only change by the power of God's saving grace, through repentance of sin, and by developing a healthy lifestyle that includes God, a healthy food plan, exercise, and a commitment to change. You have to take the first step. God's Word promises, "If you will resist the devil, he will flee from you" (James 4:7).

Lesson 4

Chef Satan's Empire of Deception
(he's the connoisseur of unhealthy eating)

Look up the dictionary definition of "chef" and write it here:

____

Now look up "connoisseur" __________________________________

And…"Satan" ____

Satan's responsibility as the "head chef" of unhealthy eating is to destroy the body by attacking every area in which we function: that includes emotionally, socially, and physically. Satan has created an epidemic through our food industry that has caused unhealthiness, obesity, and addictions, and this is now a nationwide concern. Would you agree that he is a very successful chef? He and his staff have done an excellent job.

Chefs have people who work under them to fulfill the many tasks that are required for a successful business. Whom would you say Satan employs? Am I safe to say, the one third of the angels that fell with him from the heavens? They oversee the food industry making sure it properly functions, using their creativity to develop foods that can destroy you and hold you in captivity and sin. What types of food do they oversee? JUNK!

If Satan is the connoisseur of unhealthy food, then God is the connoisseur of healthy eating. We are God's workers. He has appointed us to examine Satan's menu. God has placed us in charge of overseeing, examining, testing, and destroying Satan's menu—the one that feeds poison to God's people.

The goal for this lesson is to learn to differentiate the bad choices from the good among the vast numbers of food options. We are to make decisions on what is healthy to eat and what is not.

The result will be a healthy, personalized menu that includes foods designed to build and create high-functioning physical bodies as created and designed by God Himself. God's Word gives us clear instructions about what types of food we are to feed our body.

Read Daniel 1:3-16. "Then the king ordered Ashpenaz, who was in charge of the palace, to bring to the palace some of the young men of Judah's royal family and other noble families, who had been brought to Babylon as captive's. ' Select only strong, healthy, and good looking young men,' he said. 'Make sure they are well versed in every branch of learning, are gifted with knowledge and good sense, and have the poise needed to serve in the royal palace. Teach these young men the language and literature of Babylonians.'"

The king assigned them a daily ration of the best food and wine from his own kitchens. They were to be trained for a three-year period, and then some of them would be made his advisors in the royal court. Daniel, Hananiah, Mishael, and Azariah were four of the young men chosen.

But Daniel made up his mind not to defile himself by eating the fatty, calorie-stuffed food and wine given to them by the king. He asked the chief official for permission to eat foods allowed by Jewish law instead. Now God had given the chief official great respect for Daniel. But he was alarmed by Daniel's suggestion. "My Lord, the king, has ordered that you eat this food and wine," he said. "If you become pale and thin compared to the other youths your age, I am afraid the king will have me beheaded for neglecting my duties" (Daniel 1:10-13).

Daniel talked it over with the attendant who had been appointed by the chief official to look after him and his three friends. "Test us for ten days on a diet of vegetables and water," Daniel said. "At the end of ten days, see how we look compared to the other young men who are eating the king's rich food. Then you can decide whether or not to let us continue eating our diet" (14-16). The attendant agreed to Daniel's suggestion and tested them for the ten days. At the end of that time, Daniel and his three friends looked healthier and better nourished than the young men who had been eating the food assigned by the king. After that, the attendant fed them only vegetables instead of the rich foods and wines.

Does this mean that God wants us to limit our diet to vegetables only? Of course not.

But notice that Daniel made up his mind not to *defile himself*, and chose not to eat the king's food and drink his wine. Look up the word "defile" in your dictionary and write the definition here:

____

I like the synonym "pollute." Pollute means to make foul or corrupt. I find it interesting that Daniel recognized what the king's food and wine would do to his body. You see, Babylon was the center of pagan, ungodly civilization. The king's kitchen was being overseen by Chef Satan, and his crew was preparing the food in the palace in Babylon.

In contrast, when the children of Israel were being led out of Egypt, their kitchen was overseen by God. He personally fed them daily what their bodies required to remain healthy:

Before continuing, read Exodus chapter 16.

Even when the children of Israel wandered for forty years, God fed them. Exodus 16:13 tells us, "The next morning the desert all around the camp was wet with dew. When the dew disappeared later in the morning, thin flakes, white like frost, covered the ground."

The carnal side of me imagines those manna flakes as luscious, sweet, and dripping with hot fudge. Or maybe in the shape of a biscuit, smothered in gravy. I'll lay odds on the fact that the manna consisted of all the ingredients that our bodies need to function properly. The only change God made in the diet was when the children of Israel complained; God added quail to the menu. But I can guarantee you it wasn't deep fat fried!

Exodus chapter 16 also tells us that God rained down enough food for only one day, except on the sixth day. On the sixth day (Friday), He rained down a two-day supply so they would not need to gather on the Sabbath. Now if they tried to gather extra, in other words take more than they needed, it would spoil so they couldn't eat it.

Not surprisingly, some didn't listen, gorged themselves, and hoarded a basket or two of it until morning. By then it was full of maggots and had a terrible smell. However, the food they collected for the Sabbath did not spoil, for this was to be a day of rest from their normal daily tasks. God provided a healthy, regulated diet. No more or no less than what their bodies needed for one day.

After the desert experience, God led the next generation into the Promised Land, a land said to be "flowing with milk and honey" (Exodus 3:17). In Deuteronomy 7:13, 15, Moses said, "When you arrive in the land He swore to give your ancestors, you will have large crops of grain, grapes, olives, and great herds of cattle, sheep and goats. And the Lord will protect you from all sickness. He will not let you suffer form the terrible diseases you knew in Egypt, but He will bring them all on your enemies."

According to these verses, what are some of the foods God provided?

- ____________________
- ____________________
- ____________________
- ____________________
- ____________________
- ____________________
- ____________________
- Wait a second! Where's the double cheeseburger, fries, and chocolate milkshake? Not on God's menu?

He also promised the Israelites protection from sickness and diseases: good healthy bodies! Did Chef Satan give Daniel the same promise? ___________________________

What's it going to take for God's people to wake up and see what destruction Chef Satan is causing in our diets?

As a messenger from God, I say to Chef Satan, "Let God's people go!" Then I encourage you, the believer, to follow God, and trust Him to lead you to a healthy lifestyle change. He will rain down food from heaven for you just as He did for the children of Israel. But you have to exercise faith, obedience, and self-control, with no complaining!

Let's go grocery shopping.

Good shopping cart (foods on God's menu):

- Fresh fruit
- Fresh vegetables
- Whole-grains in breads, cereals, crackers, etc.
- Olive oil or canola oil
- Fish
- Chicken, turkey, and, yes, beef, once in a while
- Low fat milk
- Yogurt (watch for added sugars)
- Low fat cottage cheese

Yep, all the good stuff!

Bad shopping cart (foods Chef Satan wants us to eat):

- Sugar
- White flour
- Fats especially the, saturated ones
- Butter
- Fast foods
- Sodas
- Fried foods
- Pasta/white rice in excess
- Cream sauces
- Boxed dinners
- Ice cream
- Cookies, cakes, pastries
- Chips

What learn from our shopping experience? If we eat in moderation and follow a healthy diet from our good shopping cart, if we exercise and give our body plenty of rest and fluids—in other words, if we care for ourselves as we are instructed, we will reap the benefits.

Good Results
Healthiness
Weight loss
Renewed energy
Improved self-image

Now if we eat according to our bad shopping cart, we are eating a total diet prepared by Chef Satan and his crew. If we do not control that diet we will reap the results of the damage those foods cause.

Evil Results
Unhealthiness
Sickness
Disease
Obesity

Take five or ten minutes to do a quick inventory of what is in your home's refrigerator and/or pantry. Use the shopping cart lists as an easy way to check them off. This inventory will give you an idea of some of the changes you need to request to get you on the road to a healthy body.

Every person is different, but we were all fashioned by the same Creator. Even though we are all different, we were designed to eat a similar diet. Now some of us are tall, some short, there are blondes, red heads, brunettes, all types of ethnic backgrounds, some of us have small feet, some of us big feet (smile), some are large-framed or small. However, God chose to make you and me in His image, and He did not intend for us to be unhealthy!

Section 2

The Plague

Lesson 5

Steal

"The thief's purpose is to steal, and kill, and destroy" John 10:10.

What are some things Satan plans to steal?

- Our authority
- Our joy
- Our health
- Our self-control
- Our self-worth
- ____________ (add your own)
- ____________ (add your own)

This would be a good place to stop and take a personal assessment. The more honest you can be, the better, since the first step in making positive changes is acknowledging your current state of well being.

Are you happy? Yes/No
Do you frequently experience joy? Yes/No
Do you feel good? Yes/No
Do you usually have enough energy to keep going strong all day? Yes/No
Do you have great self-control? Yes/No Any self-control? Yes/No
Can you pass up second or third helpings of that favorite food? Yes/No
Can you eat a salad instead of a full meal or a hamburger and fries? Yes/No
Do you rate your self-worth as high? Yes/No
Can you truthfully stand in front of a full-length mirror and like what you see? Yes/No
Can you go shopping and purchase an article of clothing and say to yourself, I look really good in this? Yes/No

If you answered no to some or most of these questions, then Satan is stealing from you and taken over the authority in your life.

When you are caught off guard—unprepared or weak—you are vulnerable to transfer of authority. Satan will rob you of your joy, health, self-control, self-worth, and he can do this because you have given him the authority. He has stolen it from you. Get up and get your clothes back on! Gear up in your armor—your godly armor (see Ephesians 6:1-10) and take back what Satan has stolen from you. We will cover this aspect of your healthy lifestyle journey in more detail in chapter 14.

Again, regaining your authority will only come from (1) recognizing your unhealthy lifestyle as sin, (2) repenting and believing that God is faithful to forgive all sin, and then (3) beginning that healthy lifestyle change.

Lesson 6

Kill

"The thief's purpose is to steal, and kill, and destroy." (John 10:10)

What is Satan's killing plan? He tries to steal our souls, but he also tries to destroy us physically through self-abuse. Here is a list of a few of the strategies he uses.

- Cancer
- Heart disease
- Diabetes
- Mental health
- Eating disorders
- Obesity
- Addictions
- Suicide
- High blood pressure

I could write a separate book about every one of these strategies. Because of my years of obesity, I have developed a form of diabetes. Praise God, I now control that disease with a healthy diet. I told you in my introduction that I was also diagnosed with arterial inflammation, which is a heart disease. Over my lifetime, I have purged, taken powders, diet pills, experienced acupuncture in the ears (when stimulated it's supposed to send messages to your brain that you're not hungry), but none of these really solved my food addiction permanently.

Satan's attacks on our mental or emotional health are very destructive, and that strategy strikes in many different ways. It is nothing short of mental abuse, with Satan being the abuser. Some of the paths through which he chooses to attack are low self-esteem (which is a silent hell in itself), discouragement, and disgrace. All of this stress is extremely destructive, not only to your mental health, but also to your physical and social well-being. When things reach their worst point, suicide can even result. I can truthfully say that I have experienced all the phases of destruction. I know what I'm talking about. This is the reason for this book. I want to shout the message from every hilltop: There is freedom and forgiveness from The Trap, The Plague, and for The Dwelling. Praise the name of Jesus!

Read Psalm 91 and ask God to reveal His personal message to you through this Scripture. Write what you hear Him saying here or in your journal.

Lesson 7

Destroy

"The thief's purpose is to steal, and kill, and destroy." John 10:10

How does Satan destroy us?

- Through the unhealthy food choices we make and consume
- Through the way we choose to neglect our bodies by lack of exercise
- Through addictions to sugar, nicotine, illegal drugs, and alcohol
- Through our low self-esteem and lack of confidence
- Through discouragement when we fail
- ____(add your own)
- ____(add your own)

Resist the urge to make Satan the scapegoat for your sinning and failures. We are all responsible for our conscious choices. But sometimes we unknowingly make poor decisions. I am convinced and convicted by the Holy Spirit that God's people have been tricked by Satan and are sometimes blind to the destruction he has created. *He* is the reason people's health and bodies are being destroyed.

Satan is destroying us physically by the types of food we eat, the amount of food we eat, and what it does to our health. I have been concerned about and often question the ingredients in the food we buy: chemicals, sprays, preservatives, and dyes. Now we are dealing with recalls due to e-coli, melamine, as well as mad cow disease and bird flu scares. The danger of trans fat is also a huge debate in our country, and many believe that the government should intervene to prevent its use.

We willfully make decisions on a daily basis that determine what we eat, if we exercise, and if we're going to spend time with God. These decisions affect our entire body and our spirit. Disaster comes by making poor decisions.

I can try to illustrate what it felt like when God revealed the truth to me. Do you remember the old-fashioned window shades? The kind on a roller that you pulled down a little and then let go. If you weren't careful, they flew all the way up. That's what God did to my eyelids, and, when He did, the truth was brighter than the sun.

God is faithful to forgive our sins: those we willfully do and those we do unknowingly. But before He can forgive us, we have to allow ourselves to be examined by the Holy Spirit to convict us of our sin. By use of our conscience, He can help us to know when we have done something wrong. Satan has been so clever regarding our health that I am convinced many people are in the same condition I was before the shades flew up: blinded from the truth. I truly believe people do not recognize unhealthiness as sin. I encourage you to examine your heart, and turn from the sin you have committed against your body, and then do something to change. God will help you.

Lesson 8

Good vs. Evil

Look up the key Scriptures below and write them out in the space provided:

1 John 5:19 ____

____

John 8:44 ____

____

____

According to these Scriptures, what words characterize Satan?

____

Since God's Word is final, it's safe to say Satan is the ruler of our world as we know it. So what has he ever done to make it a better place in which to live? Remember: he's a liar and he is out to kill, steal, and destroy (John 10:10).

Being unhealthy could be termed Satan's hell on earth. What a master plan he has developed! Christians everywhere have swallowed his plan hook, line and sinker! An unhealthy diet creates total havoc and chaos within your body. Diseases attack every working cell, muscle, joint, and organ of your body from your head down to your feet.

But *why* does the food we eat cause obesity and unhealthiness? The medical experts, nutritionists, schools, the media—all express concern about the problems our food is causing. Books have been written, diet programs have been formulated, and our food industry claims to support a healthy lifestyle. So why do people continue to have grave physical problems? From senior citizens to pre-born infants—unhealthiness is an epidemic.

As I began to research the medical explanations for how our bodies are designed and should work, the contrast between who I was and who I should be was so great that I fell to my knees before God and asked for His forgiveness. I realized that I had abused the body He so wonderfully made.

Psalm 139:14 ____

Ephesians 2:10: ____

2 Corinthians 7:1 ____

God began to show me that I can have victory and authority over my spiritual being AND I can have victory and authority over my physical one as well. I also saw a pattern in the similarities between the spiritual and physical victories. God began to show me that people generally view Satan as "destroying us" instantaneously, (example: car wrecks, accidents). But, I understood that Satan destroys us daily, bit by bit, and in my opinion, destruction by degrees is much more effective. It's almost an "in God's face! Ha! Ha! Ha!" because the majority of God's people won't use their spiritual armor and authority to put Satan in his place.

In Mark 7:18-20 Jesus asked, "Can't you see that what you eat won't defile you? Food doesn't come in contact with your heart, but only passes through the stomach and then comes out again." By saying this, He showed that the food itself is not sin. In reality, every kind of food is "acceptable." And then He added, "It is the thought-life that defiles you." Remember *defile* means: To pollute, or make filthy.

We as Christians are responsible to a higher standard of living—God's standard. We need to use wisdom concerning our diet so that we can become aware of what is in our food, how much of it we eat, and what it does to us. Again, food in itself is not a sin ... gluttony is...being unhealthy is. When we are following God's design for our body, we will naturally eat accordingly. Satan's diet does not contain anything healthy for us. He is out to steal, kill, and destroy.

The "heart" of my being is not the organ that pumps blood through my body. Who I am—my soul (mind, will emotions)—is actually in the center of my brain. Our brain delegates everything our body does. Located in the center of the brain is the hypothalamus. I like to think of the hypothalamus as my "sacred garden." And hidden in that garden area is the satiety center that regulates appetite, or more specifically, suppresses the desire for food when stimulated. The satiety center is controlled by two counterbalancing chemicals that are located side by side. These chemicals play an important part in how we will find victory in the battle for our health. They are the following:

- Leptin: (comes for the Greek word for thin) is a protein secreted by stored fat. It shuts off the hunger signals to the brain and stimulates you to burn more calories by stimulating CART (Cocaine and Amphetamine Regulated Transcript).
- Ghrelin: (I call it gremlin) When your stomach is empty, hormones release a chemical called Ghrelin. When your stomach is growling, it's this hormone controlling your body's offensive team. Ghrelin makes you want to eat by stimulating NPY (neuropeptide-Y, another protein.)

CART stimulates the hypothalamus to increase your metabolism, aids in reducing your appetite, and increases insulin to help deliver much needed energy to your muscle cells rather than being stored as fat. NPY decreases or slows down your metabolism, thus increasing your appetite.

One way to think of these two controlling chemicals in your body is to compare them to any team sport, such as football, basketball, or soccer. The offense is always trying to make advances, score points, plan the attack. While the defense does what? Protects its territory! If you can become aware of how your body and your mind actually work together to control what you eat, you will naturally (God's way) achieve your ideal "playing" weight.

You do this by developing a well-trained defense. Begin recognizing the Traps and the Plagues and how they affect your Dwelling. Think about what you eat. By working on this lifestyle change, you will naturally balance the offense. And by doing this, you become the winner (in the diet game) every single time. That's why it is so important to understand that

CART/Leptin (God's way)

NPY/Ghrelin (Satan's way)

are the key biological factors in regulating our health.

Have the window shades rolled up yet? Are you as excited as I was when God revealed the truth to me? Now read carefully. In your sacred garden live both CART and NPY. *You* make the decisions that allow them to function. Are you hearing me? These two body chemicals determine whether you are going to eat a truckload or eat smart by influencing the hormone that tells you if you are full or hungry. This is where the battle begins! You have a good chemical and a bad chemical and, in one sense, they help control your daily decision to eat healthily or unhealthily. What you need to do is stimulate CART through

Leptin. By keeping our Leptin levels high and our Ghrelin/NPY levels non-functioning, good defeats evil.

A few years ago, I heard a message on faith. The pastor was teaching that "the weapons of our warfare are not carnal." Your mind is the primary target Satan shoots at, and your specific thought processes comprise the bull's eye. As you retrain your mind from always thinking about food to hardly ever thinking about it, you also will be on the road to reprogramming your body. It will no longer be your eyes, tongue, mouth (as in pizza, hamburgers, sodas, and constant junk food) that will control your health. The natural chemicals in your body will be in control. When you're becoming healthy, you will understand that when your stomach growls, the chemical NPY is at work, and that cravings for healthy foods are signals from CART. Over time, you will have fewer giant cravings for junk foods and more cravings for healthy alternatives.

Section 3
The Dwelling

Lesson 9

God's Temple, Our Body

Second Corinthians 6:14-18 reads, "Don't team up with those who are unbelievers. How can goodness be a partner with wickedness? How can light live with darkness? What harmony can there be between Christ and the devil? How can a believer be a partner with an unbeliever? And what union can there be between God's temple and idols? For we are the temple of the living God. As God said, 'I will live in them and walk among them. I will be their God and they will be my people. Therefore come out from them and separate yourselves from them,' says the Lord. 'Don't touch their filthy things and I will welcome you. And I will be your Father. And you will be my sons and daughters,' says the Lord Almighty."

Find 2 Corinthians 7:1 and write it out here:

____

____

____

Notice that God speaks individually to our *body* and our *spirit*. He tells us to cleanse our body and spirit. By not caring for our body, we are living in rebellion and disobedience to what God's Word tells us to do.

I believe we can apply this Scripture, not only to our spiritual life, but to our physical one as well. A close Christian friend once said, "If sin wasn't so much fun, people wouldn't do it!" I believe this holds true with food as well. Medical experts have proven that the moment food enters our mouth, we determine where it will go and how our body will use it, according to our needs. What we choose to eat makes the resulting effect positive or negative. I challenge you to not only guard what comes out of your mouth, but what goes in it as well.

In sermons past, I have been cautioned that one of the most destructive tools Satan uses is our tongues.

Look up the dictionary definition of "the tongue" and write it here:

____

Do you realize the same tongue that can destroy people with words also controls our sense of taste, which, in a sense, determines what and how much we want to eat? Stop and think before you take that first bite: is this food good for me or bad for me? You willfully make that decision, whether you stop to think about it or not. Am I trying to apply guilt? Absolutely not! But your physical body should not be treated any differently than your spiritual body. Sin is sin.

All through the Bible, people who obeyed and trusted God were victorious in battle. God never allowed them to be defeated, but the moment sin and rebellion entered the camp, God lifted His hand of protection. God will address rebellion and disobedience. He's a good parent, and rebellion and disobedience are unacceptable behavior in children. (See Hebrews 12:6-12).

Colossians 1:13-14 reads, "For He *has* rescued us from the one who rules in the kingdom of darkness, and He *has* brought us into the Kingdom of His dear Son. God *has* purchased our freedom with His blood, and *has* forgiven all our sins." Notice the word *has*; God used it four times! The meaning of "has" is past tense! He's already done it!

Second Corinthians 4:8-10 reads, "We are pressed on every side by troubles, but we are not crushed and broken. We are perplexed (troubled) but we don't give up and quit. We are hunted down, but God never abandons us. We get knocked down, but we get up again and keep going. Through suffering, these bodies of ours constantly share in the death of Jesus, so that the life of Jesus may also be seen in our bodies."

How does this verse speak to you today regarding your battle to live a healthy lifestyle?

____

____

____

Lesson 10

Caring for the Temple

Ephesians 2:10: "For we are God's masterpiece."

1 Corinthians 9:27: "I discipline my body like an athlete, training it to do what it should."

Psalms 127:3: "Children are a gift from the Lord. They are a reward from Him."

I love babies! My mind is full of awe at the mystery of a tiny sperm cell finding its way to that perfect egg cell, and initiating the beautiful creation of a baby.

Moms are the heart of the family. Their God-ordained duty is to care for their children, both spiritually and physically, from the moment God unites that excited little sperm with that perfect little egg.

Many of today's studies show many diseases begin attacking and seeking to destroy a baby's health while the infant is still in the womb. Satan declares war on healthy babies through the abuse of alcohol, drugs, nicotine, and/or an inadequate diet.

Parents are expected to love, care, and nurture you according to God's holy Word. That's a huge responsibility for parents. Christian parents may take you to church, summer camp, and youth conventions. They may guard what you read, watch on TV, with whom you play, what movies you watch. Christian education/home schooling has become a viable and common alternative to the public school system. We have videos and books written to educate us on home life, sex, avoiding strangers, and making right choices about drugs and alcohol use. But what baffles me is how Christians can stampede to those fast food drive-up windows, stuff themselves with pizza, hotdogs, hamburgers, fat-stuffed meats, and substitute healthy foods for unhealthy ones. We replace water with sodas and sweetened drinks. We eat just about anything we want with no boundaries as to portion size.

We start our day with breakfast. Well, some of us do. Most kids grow up eating sugar-packed cereals. We have convenience foods for breakfast too: frozen pancakes (even chocolate chip!), waffles, French toast, pop-tarts, donuts, and biscuits. All quick and easy, loaded with calories, fat (saturated or hydrogenated fat), sugar (refined sugar), and practically devoid of food value.

Lunch isn't much better. We pack soft drinks, conveniently packaged chips, cookies, crackers, snack bars (most of which aren't healthy). Again, foods containing sugar (bad sugar), fat (bad fat), calories, and little or no nutritional value.

Dinner time. Most moms have worked all day, so something quick and easy usually fits most menus. Casseroles, spaghetti, frozen pizza, macaroni and cheese, hot dogs, or maybe just a quick run through the drive-up window of your favorite fast-food restaurant. Or better yet, just order in for delivery! These meals are high in fat and carbs, preservatives and salt. A recipe for obesity.

If left to fend for ourselves, our snack choices are usually unhealthy—chips, cookies, etc. And don't forget that bowl of ice cream before bedtime.

Rarely do you see bowls of fruit or little packages of prepared veggies in the fridge along with yogurt, cheese, turkey, or anything that says "good for you!" Now if your mom is one who takes the time and effort to create these healthy snacks, I salute her! If not, you may need to sit down with your mom, tell about this course you're taking, and ask how she can help. I can almost guarantee that she will respond positively! Your temple is worth caring for.

Proverbs 24:5 says: ____

____

____

____

God's Word is a constant reminder; in all situations, the first thing we are to do is seek wisdom. We are to pray, seek God's will, and realize He is faithful to answer us through godly wisdom from His Word.

During struggles and hardships, we seek counsel from our pastors, peers, financial advisors, youth leaders. When we are not feeling well we visit our family doctor, dentist, and if we are in need of glasses we seek a trusted eye doctor. God has placed good people in all of these professions, and if they are true followers of Christ, prayer will be one of the "prescriptions" recommended for healing and restoration. I am here to guide you to a healthier lifestyle. And I am praying for you!

Lesson 11

Discipline

Hebrews 12:6–13: "For the Lord disciplines those He loves, and He punishes those He accepts as his children. As you endure this divine discipline, remember that God is treating you as his own children. Whoever heard of a child who was never disciplined? If God doesn't discipline you as he does all of his children, it means you are illegitimate and are not really his after all. Since we respect our earthly fathers who disciplined us, should we not all the more cheerfully submit to the discipline of our heavenly Father and live forever? For our earthly fathers disciplined us for a few years, doing the best they knew how. But God's discipline is always right and good for us because it means we will share in his holiness. No discipline is enjoyable while it is happening—it is painful! But afterward there will be a quiet harvest of right living for those who are trained in this way. So take a new grip with your tired hands and stand firm on your shaky legs. Mark out a straight path for your feet. Then those who follow you, though they are weak and lame, will not stumble and fall but will become strong."

Revelation 3:19 is brief and to the point. Write it out here:

____

Who is speaking in this verse? ____

Look up the word "discipline" in your dictionary and write it here:

____

____

Discipline, as you now can see, is not punishment. Discipline involves training. What are a few ways we can discipline (train) ourselves to eat healthily? ____________________

____

What should the training of discipline produce?

____

How can we exercise self-control (will power, determination, or drive)? By following a system—just like an athlete follows a regimen to keep in shape and improve his or her skills. A system provides direction, guidelines, even commands to ensure the optimum result.

In our journey to be fit for life, we need to discipline (train) ourselves to seek wisdom and knowledge from God's Word. We can accomplish this by training ourselves to be obedient in daily devotions—spending time alone with God. We must pray each day. In this way, we'll begin recognizing God's voice when He speaks to us, and being obedient, we will listen.

We also need to train ourselves to recognize the influence of our food choices, and consciously make healthy choices. This training requires perseverance and self-control. (See Romans 5:3, 4 and James 1:3-5.) To have self-control you need will power; from will power, you develop determination and drive.

A good system includes techniques (guidelines) to follow. Here are some that have been useful for me:

1. Using 3x5 index cards, write down four or five Scriptures that deal with the problem you are facing. (Examples: self-control, temptation, discipline, obedience), and read them aloud with conviction. Use your authority and put Satan in his place. Take his power away from him. Recognize he is POWERLESS in comparison to Christ!

2. Set achievable goals. Place a mental picture of who you are in Christ, and then guard that picture with your Scripture cards. You are in spiritual warfare.

3. Think about CART and NPY and which one of them you want to rule over your food choices.

4. Decide on your style of diet, plan your method, and engage your system. Develop a support group, help your mom plan grocery shopping, and do prep work. Have a strategy for success.

Some Tips for you and your mom:

- Before you shop or go to a gathering where there will be food, pray and ask God for self-control.
- While you are facing an eating situation—party, restaurant, visiting amusement park or mall, friend's house—pray for God to remove the temptations.
- Keep your Leptin levels high by eating healthy foods (see God's shopping cart in chapter X).
- Pray without ceasing, sing praises, TALK to yourself, well, to God. It works!

5. Exercise: Begin walking a mile a day, or play tennis, or use an exercise machine—whatever you enjoy or feel capable of doing. Over time, these things will become natural for you. The direction or path you have marked out for your shaky legs will start out as tiny steps and end in a run with the Lord. Your need for determination, drive, self-control, will power, and obedience will become subject to your system of rules if you are consistent and rely on God's wisdom to sustain you.

Karate Kid: Wax On, Wax Off

Do you remember the classic movie: The Karate Kid? If not, briefly, the plot is about a boy in high school named Daniel who is bullied by boys who know karate. Daniel meets an elderly Japanese man, Mr. Miyagi, who used to be a karate master. He calls Daniel *Daniel-san* and agrees to begin training him, but his training methods are strange. He begins by making Daniel wax his cars, sand down a deck, paint a fence, keep his balance on one leg in crashing waves—hard work that seemingly has no connection at all to karate training. However, without knowing it, Daniel-san is gaining strength and stamina, learning discipline, patience, and self-control, and catching on to important karate skills. All of this takes place through sweat, physical labor, and an inner determination to succeed.

Daniel-san's situation:
#1 His problem: Daniel-san didn't recognize the teaching, because he couldn't see past the work.
#2 His response: He complained to his master.
#3 His threat: He finally exploded and claimed he would quit.

Our situation:

#1 Our problem: Sometimes we can't see the solutions because we can't look past the present and believe in the unknown

#2 So what do we do? We complain to the Master

#3 We want to quit.

After Mr. Miyagi showed Daniel the importance behind all of the work he was doing, he understood and then received Knowledge, Wisdom, and Understanding.

Mr. Miyagi possessed great wisdom. He knew when Daniel-san was ready for competition before Daniel knew it. When Mr. Miyagi accepted the challenge for the first Karate match, the training time followed.

Mr. Miyagi found favor in Daniel-san and rewarded him for all his hard labor with one of his own vintage cars for his sixteenth birthday. Over time, mutual love, respect, and friendship developed as a special bond between the master and his student.

God used this movie as an illustration of His relationship with me—that although I sometimes say I'm willing and eager to do the right thing, I must also have the willingness to be taught by a patient and loving Master. This teaching will come through my obedience, discipline, and hard work, which is the exact recipe for moving from being unhealthy to healthy.

I recommend you rent "Karate Kid" and watch it again through the eyes of your newfound wisdom about discipline. See if you are inspired and encouraged as I was. Record your thoughts and ideas in your journal.

Lesson 12

Personal Responsibility

Read and write out the following Scriptures carefully. They contain the secret to success in your battle to be healthy.

Proverbs 4:20-22: ____

____

____

Proverbs 4:23: ____

____

Proverbs 4:25: ____

____

____

Do not let your tummy's growls tempt you to grab for junk food every time you want to chomp on something. (Remember the gremlin Grehlin.) Life and radiant health comprise two completely different promises. The promise of radiant health is to anyone who discovers its meaning.

Life = Active principle of existence

Radiant health = Beaming, shining, emitting rays, soundness of body, a well-conditioned body.

Proverbs 4:34 says to guard your heart. This is poetic language for guarding your soul, which includes your mind (your sacred garden). Remember it's the thought life that defiles you. You can control what you think, and that includes your food choices and what you eat. Remember the two chemicals, NPY and CART? CART being the positive chemical and NPY being the negative chemical. You have the power through your choices as to which one of these chemicals will win the battle going on within your body chemistry.

It is difficult for us to accept the fact that friends, acquaintances, and even family may lure us to do wrong. While we should be accepting of others, we need a healthy skepticism regarding whether we should always copy what they do; we need a healthy skepticism about human behavior. When you feel yourself being heavily influenced, proceed with caution. Don't let your friends cause you to do what is wrong for you.

Proverbs 4:25, above, emphasized our need to prepare our minds with an image of who we are, and who we want to be. You can prepare your mind by:

- Planning your strategy
- Deciding daily what you are going to eat.
- Being prepared in advance.
- Not straying from your plan.

Are you always going to eat the right thing? Probably not, but recognize your weakness as wrong, quit it, and get back on track. Walk an extra twenty or thirty minutes to burn off the extra calories, and keep pressing forward. Over time, you will retrain your mind and body to do and eat what is right for you. Always "run toward the prize," and you'll win in the long run.

Romans 12:1-2, "And so dear brothers and sisters, I plead with you to give your bodies to God. Let them be a living and holy sacrifice... the kind He will accept. When you think of what He has done for you, is this too much to ask? Don't copy the *behavior* and *customs* of this world, but let God transform you into a new person by changing the way you think. Then you will know what God wants you to do and you will know how good and pleasing and perfect His will really is."

Look up the following words in your dictionary:

Behaviors: ____

Customs or habits: ____

What ungodly behaviors, customs, or habits of the World have you been imitating?

____

____

____

As God's messenger, I give each of you this word of advice:

1. Be honest in your estimate of yourself, measuring your value by how much faith God has given you.

Your value is your worth and your importance. Your faith is your trust in God, your decision to believe, even without proof, and your loyalty to Him and His Word.

2. Just as our bodies have many parts and each part has a special function, so it is with Christ's body. We are all parts of His one body, and each of us has a different work to do. And since we are all one body in Christ, we belong to each other, and each of us needs all the others. (Read 1 Corinthians 12:12 and Romans 12.)

Check out the important Scriptures below. Read them a couple of times.

Romans 14:10, "So why do you condemn another Christian. Why do you look down on another Christian? Remember, each of us will stand personally before the judgment seat of God. For the Scriptures say, 'As surely as I live,' says the Lord, 'Every knee will bow to me and every tongue will confess allegiance to God.' "

What do you think the word "condemn" means? ______________________________

What does "judging" mean? ______________________________

Who judges us on earth? ______________________________

Why? ______________________________

Who is the ultimate judge of our hearts? ______________________________

Romans 14:13, "Yes, each of us will have to give a personal account to God. So don't condemn each other anymore. Decide instead to live in such a way that you will not put an obstacle in another Christian's path."

Romans 14:14, "I know and am perfectly sure on the authority of the Lord Jesus Christ that no food, in and of itself, is wrong to eat. But if someone believes it is wrong, then for that person it is wrong. And if another Christian is distressed by what you eat, you are not acting in love if you eat it. Don't let your eating ruin someone for whom Christ died. Then you will not be condemned for doing something you know is right. For the Kingdom of God is not a matter of what we eat or drink, but of living a life of goodness and peace and joy in the Holy Spirit. If you serve Christ with this attitude, you will please God. And other people will approve of you too. So, then let us aim for harmony in the church and try to build each other up.

"Don't tear apart the work of God over what you eat. Remember, there is nothing wrong with these things in themselves. But, it is wrong to eat anything if it makes another person stumble. You may have the faith to believe that there is nothing wrong with what you are doing, but keep it between yourself and God. Blessed are those who do not condemn themselves by doing something they know is right. But if people have doubts about whether they should eat something, they shouldn't eat it. They would be condemned for not acting in faith before God. If you do anything you believe is not right, you are sinning."

I have to ask you, and please answer this question honestly. Do you believe it is okay to eat and drink whatever you want with no restrictions? Do you believe it's okay not to exercise? Do you believe it is okay for you and your family to live in an unhealthy environment? God's Word teaches us that we are to care for our temple bodies. Remember, I'm not the big authority here, I'm just the messenger. He says that if we do anything we believe is not right, we are *sinning*. As a child of God, you cannot say unhealthiness is right! Unhealthiness is 100 percent against God's Word.

We try to steer clear of actions forbidden by Scripture, but sometimes Scripture is silent. In those cases, we should follow our conscience: "If you do anything you believe is not right, you are sinning." This means that to go against a conviction will leave a person with a guilty or uneasy conscience. When God shows us something is wrong for us, we should avoid it.

Is God convicting you of something you have been doing (or not doing) or eating (or not eating) that you know is wrong? Write it down here or in your journal. Confess it to Him, repent, and begin now to avoid this behavior, to the glory of God!

Section 4
Freedom from Sin's Grasp

Lesson 13

Taking Authority

Webster's dictionary defines "authority" as: ______________________________

____

Let's talk about authority, what it is and what it means.

Matthew 28:18 (Jesus speaking): "I have been given complete authority in Heaven and on Earth." Jesus tells us that He has been given authority, which means assigned power, transfer of power, and/or delegated power. The Father transferred this authority to His Son. Then in Luke 10:19, the Son (Jesus) gives *us* that same authority (which is God's assigned power), over the power of the enemy.

Think about God's power. This power causes the earth to tremble, volcanoes to erupt, tidal waves to crush, the stars to fall from the sky. This same power speaks to the storms and says, "Peace, be still." God created the sun to rise for daylight and the moon to shine at night. This same power was transferred to His Son, and His Son transferred that power to those whose names are written in the Lamb's Book of Life. This authority was given to us in order to crush Satan and all his works.

Satan is powerless against you! Jesus said in Luke 10:19, "I have given you authority over all the power of the enemy and you can walk among snakes and scorpions and crush them."

Look up the following verses and write them in the space provided:

Ephesians 1:19: ____

____

____

Ephesians 2:4-6 ____

____

____

1Peter 5:8 ____

____

____

Satan is called by many different names in Scripture: Prince of this world, Father of Lies, Accuser, Lucifer, Beelzebub, the Devil, Angel of Light, the Evil One. In the verse you wrote above, he is compared to a lion.

Lions attack because it is part of their nature. Likewise, Satan's nature, because of his rebellion against God, has no pity or genuine love of any kind. Lions will search for the weak, sick, young, or struggling—-those who are alone or are not alert. He detects them, stalks them, intimidates them, and makes the prey aware of his presence. Then, in a flash, the lion moves in for the kill with speed, agility, and determination to destroy.

Many types of animals stay together in groups (herds, flocks, etc.) to protect themselves from predators. At least one animal is always on the lookout for danger and warns the rest of the herd that danger is near. When the herd makes their run to escape from danger, this is when the unprepared, sick, weak, ones are taken down. Whatever is stalking this herd has already figured out which ones are weak. They are his target.

Peter warns us to watch out for Satan when we are suffering or persecuted. When we're feeling alone, weak, helpless, and cut off from other believers, we become so focused on our troubles that we forget to watch for danger. We are especially vulnerable to Satan's attacks. . Keep your eyes on Christ and resist the Devil. Then says James, "he will flee from you" (James 4:7).

During times of suffering or weakness, seek other Christians for support. Keep your eyes on Christ. Form walking clubs and accountability groups or partners. Have weekly meetings of teaching and encouragement. Pray! Pray! Pray! Read God's Word, meditate on every word. Sing praises to the Lord. Train your mind to focus on God moment by moment.

When that temptation closes in, PRAY. Remove yourself from the situation, exercise will power, call your prayer partner, do whatever is necessary to force your body into submission. Remember who is in control. This is a battle for your health. Resist the devil and he will flee from you!

If you follow this plan, you will begin having small victories over your temptation. Allowing God to have your anxieties calls for action, not passivity. Don't submit to circumstances, but to the Lord, who controls our circumstances.

Unhealthy Christians have given transfer of power (authority) of our bodies over to Satan. He is caring for the body God intended for us to protect. Maybe you've heard the saying, "So-and-so is eating their lunch." Well, if you're destroying your body, "Satan's eating your lunch!" I challenge you to say instead, "I'm "eating Satan's lunch," and lots of it." (And by this, I don't mean eating Chef Satan's menu!) Food is everywhere we look. We need to recognize that this is one of the most tempting traps Satan has set. Romans 12:2 says, "Don't copy the behavior and customs of this world, but let God transform you into a new person by changing the way you think."

We recognize pornography, sexual immorality, homosexuality, abortion, and corruption as sin. Unhealthy foods and the lifestyle that accompanies them are also sins. We as believers need to rise up and take back our authority! Satan can only control what authority we give him. DON'T GIVE HIM ANY. Use your authority and break those food addictions. Reclaim your health and begin treating your body the way God instructed you to. We need to realize who we are in Christ. We need to be in Christ (born again) to have the authority. We can't be in a hurry to fight battles. The CART vs. NPY battles are won and lost in the mind (your sacred garden). Spiritual battling (warfare) requires the Word of God. The Word of God is your victory banner. We need to understand the power we have in Christ and turn off the source of power coming from Satan. Remind yourself that he is powerless.

"He who is in you is greater than he who is in the world" (1 John 4:4 NKJV).

Lesson 14

Putting on the Armor

In Ephesians 6:10-12, we learn that how to protect ourselves from Satan's Traps. "Put on all of God's armor so that you will be able to stand firm against all the strategies, and tricks of the Devil. For we are not fighting against people made of flesh and blood, but against the evil rulers and authorities of the unseen world, against those mighty powers of darkness who rule this world, and against the wicked spirits in the heavenly realms" (a.k.a. Chef Satan). "Use every piece of God's armor to resist the enemy in the time of evil, so that after the battle you will be standing firm."

According to verses 13 through 17 what are the pieces of this armor?

The ______________ of ______________

The ______________ of ______________

The ______________ of ______________

The ______________ of ______________

The ______________ of ______________

The ______________ of ______________

The armor of God is our garment of protection in war. He has clothed us from head to toe. Before any battle, you have to be properly trained. Then you are fitted with your armor of protection, custom made, just for you.

When soldiers go to war, they set up camp and, then set up perimeters of safety around the camp. As believers doing warfare against Satan, we also need to set up perimeters. Your eye gate, ear gate, and your mouth gate need to be guarded. Everything that attempts to go through these gates needs to be examined: the food you see, the food you hear about, and the food you eat. When you put on your spiritual armor and use your spiritual weapons, strongholds will be destroyed. You will be set FREE!

Proverbs 24:6 says:

____

I believe healthiness falls under the subject of spiritual warfare, and God's Word prepares us for that battle. When you realize the stronghold Satan has over you regarding your health, you as a believer have no choice but to go to war.

So how do we prepare for the battle?

1. Seek God in prayer
2. Study His Word, the Bible.
3. Learn how He designed our bodies and how they function (strategy)
4. Dress yourself with your armor of protection
5. With orders in hand, report to your leading commander

Our leading commander is God and His Word. God has also strategically placed other believers to help us as we fulfill our work here on Earth. God will direct your path as long as He is the one leading the way. (See Proverbs 3:5-6).

As we learned in lesson 1, the first step toward victory is repentance. You have to recognize unhealthiness as sin. When you do, your strategy for war will be successful. I cannot emphasize repentance enough. If you will grab onto God's Word, the truth will set you free. If you sin, repent and sin no more! Healthiness will follow, but you have to be the one to make the change. When you do your part, God will do His part. James 4:17 reads, "It is a sin to know what you ought to do, and then not do it." What does this Scripture tell us to do? It tells us to repent. And if we know we should be doing something, and aren't doing it, we're living in sin. So my conclusion is: if you know you're unhealthy, overweight, guilty of abusing your body through addictions, lack of exercise, and aren't doing anything to change that lifestyle, you are sinning. God's Word tells us to care for both our physical and spiritual bodies. The only way we're going to succeed and overcome the sin in our lives is through repentance. John 8:11 "Go and sin no more."

Lesson 15

How to Recognize Satan's Voice

Do my ideas agree with the Word of God? Are you willing to change your habits? Are you being tempted to eat a food you know is not healthy? We need to train our bodies to really listen. God speaks to us all the time, and He has designed our bodies to speak to us in the same way. Our body tells us when it's hungry, thirsty, tired, sad, happy, depressed, angry, and in pain. We need to identify what our bodies are telling us regarding the care and health of our body. Examine every temptation or craving you sense. Is the choice good for you or bad for you? Is CART at work? Or is NPY having its way?

James 4:7 says: "So humble yourselves before God, resist the devil and he will flee from you!" Why are you overweight? Why do you overeat? Do you lack self-control and will power? We seem to have no authority over the type of food we eat or how much we eat. We need to recognize the problem and fix it. The problem is sin. So if the problem is sin, what's the solution? Repentance! You have to make the decision to change your physical lifestyle. You have the power to control what and how much you eat.

Pick up your sword (the Word of God) and make the necessary lifestyle changes to win the battle. You need to take back your authority from Satan. You have a free will to sin or not to sin. The battle involves the destruction of your health (Satan's way) vs. the freedom to be healthy (God's way).

Satan is a Liar and a Thief!

In John 8:44, Jesus said, "He (Satan) was a murderer from the beginning and has always hated the truth. There is no truth in him. When he lies, it is consistent with his character; for he (Satan) is a liar and the father of lies."

Then Paul added in 2 Corinthians 10: 3-4, "We are human, but we do not wage war with human plans and methods. We use God's mighty weapons, not mere worldly weapons to knock down the devil's strongholds." God's Word tells us to bring every

THOUGHT into CAPTIVITY (2 Corinthians 10:5 NKJV) and CONTROL it. That should include every bite of food as well. Put up your STOP sign and stop Satan. Who is standing guard at your mouth gate and in your sacred garden that is located in the center of your brain?

Lesson 16

Sin's Power is Broken

My ambition is to preach the Word in a way that people have never heard, rather than where a church has already been started by someone else. Just as Paul, a Jew, was called to preach the good news to the Gentiles, so am I being called to preach the good news to God's chosen people. God is going to show them there is power in the name (authority) of Jesus. They are not powerless.

When food, discouragement, failure, the inability to exercise, or anything else gets us down, we need to stop and make the decision not to give in to that feeling. Instead, shout: "I have authority! There is power in the name of Jesus!" You only need to speak it once. You have the power! It was given to you by Christ. Satan has no power or authority. He lies to you and makes you believe he is unbeatable. He is not! He is power-less with Jesus at your side!

I repeat, sin's power is broken. Romans 6:12-14 reads, "Do not let sin control the way you live, do not give in to its lustful desires. Do not let any part of your body become a tool of wickedness to be used for sinning. Instead, give yourselves completely to God since you have been given new life. And use your whole body as a tool to do what is right for the glory of God. Sin is no longer your master, for you are no longer subject to the laws which enslave you to sin. Instead, you are free by God's grace."

The scripture says, "Do not let sin control the way you live. Again, what is sin? Look the word up in your dictionary.

Sin: ____

____

If we have died to sin, how can we continue to live in it? When we became Christians, we became one with Christ. We died with Him. Since we have been united with Him in

His death, we will also be raised with Him. Our old sinful lives were crucified with Christ so that sin would lose its power in our lives. We are no longer slaves to sin. Look up and write out the following two verses about the sinful nature:

Romans 8:7: ____

Romans 8:5: ____

____

____

Romans 6:12 says, "Do not give in to *its* lustful desires." What is "its" in the statement above? ____

Right! Do not give in to *sin's* lustful desires. And what is the meaning of lust? Look up the word in your dictionary and write out the definitions here: ______________________

____

____

Apply this to what you eat. What do you lust for? List your cravings:

____

____

____

Romans 6: 13: "Do not let any part of your body become a tool of wickedness to be used for sinning."

Look up the definition of tool: ______________________________

Look up the definition of wickedness: __________________________

____

Wyndy's definition of "tool of wickedness" is this: An evil contraption (the tongue) that is an appliance for mechanical operations (your eating). Remember this the next time you make the decision to eat that greasy hamburger or that triple scoop ice cream cone.

Romans 6:12 says, "Whatever you choose to *obey* becomes your master."

Obey means to do as ordered, submit to authority, and follow.

You can choose sin, which leads to death, or you can choose to obey God and receive His approval. Approval is His blessing, His endorsement. Even better than a vintage car. Our Master gives eternal life.

Paul uses the example of slaves and masters to demonstrate freedom vs. bondage. "But now you are free from the power of sin and have become slaves of God. Now you do those things that lead to holiness and eternal life" (healthiness).

Then in 1 Corinthians 6:9 we read, "Don't you know that those who do wrong will have no share in the kingdom of God? Don't fool yourselves. Those who indulge in sexual sin, who are idol worshipers, adulterers, male prostitutes, homosexuals, thieves, *greedy people,* drunkards, *abusers,* and swindlers – none of these will have a share in the Kingdom of God."

Let's examine some of these people who will not be a part of God's kingdom.

Greedy people: those who indulge in excessive consumption of, or desire for, food; wealth.

Abusers: misusers of something or someone (including self)

This stings a bit, doesn't it? But often the truth is what sets us free. I know it set me free.

Controlling the Tongue and what we stuff into the Mouth

James 3:2ff: "We all make many mistakes, *but those who control their tongues can also control themselves in every other way.* We can make a large horse turn around and go wherever we want by means of a small bit in its mouth, and a tiny rudder makes a huge ship turn wherever the pilot wants it to go even though the winds are strong. So also the tongue is a small thing, but what enormous damage it can do. A tiny spark can set a great forest on fire, and the tongue is a flame of fire. It is full of wickedness that can ruin your whole life. It can turn the entire course of your life into a blazing flame of destruction, for it is set on fire by hell itself."

Medical research claims the tongue to be the most powerful muscle in the body, and in more way than one, it wields power. God's Word tells us how destructive our tongue is spiritually because of things we say to others. A second major function of the tongue is for tasting food. The tongue tastes with papillae that sense chemicals in foods, and tell you whether they're worth your attention. If not carefully examined by you, that is a dangerous journey for your body! If you eat everything that looks like it might taste good, you're going to be as big as a house.

Our bodies use our senses to process information. We depend on our tongue to instruct us on food. The instruction or information we receive sends messages to our brain (our secret garden). Our brain then speaks to our forks. Keep eating or stop eating. A large part of this message comes from our five taste senses: sweet, sour, salty, bitter, umami (recognizes freshness and "tastiness").

Well, how do we tame our tongue in regard to food? "Whatsoever things are…?" healthy, good for you, small in portion, under the authority of God's Word, controlled.

Romans 6:23, "For the wages of sin is death, but the free gift of God is eternal life through Christ Jesus our Lord." In Romans 7:18-25, Paul explains his struggle with sin. Read these verses then apply to your struggle with eating healthy foods. Do you have:

Temptation for great amounts of food?

Temptation for junk with no nutritional value?

Lack of desire for exercise?

Lack of will power?

Where's the answer? In Christ Jesus our Lord! So you see how it is. In my mind, I really want to obey God's law, but because of my sinful nature, I am a slave to sin. God destroyed sin's control over us by giving us His Son as a sacrifice for our sin. Those who are dominated by the sinful nature think about sinful things, but those who are controlled by the Holy Spirit think about things that please God. If your sinful nature controls your mind, there is death. But if the Holy Spirit controls your mind, there is life and peace. Freedom. Health.

Conclusion

I'm Convinced! Now What?

There! Can you believe you're almost done with this course? Maybe you feel hope and you've already kicked off the beginning of a new lifestyle. On the other hand, maybe you feel discouraged and hopeless, or maybe you have a simmering anger toward me for making you feel guilty. Please don't give up, and don't be mad at God because of me. After all, God is the One who says you're a temple He wants to lives in, and He wants that temple to be first class and running at top efficiency. I'm just the messenger.

Is food sinful? Is enjoying a fabulous meal wrong? Of course not. Food and enjoying food are gifts from God. I've been tough on you because if you're overweight, unhealthy, sickly, or out of shape, it means you've been badly abusing the gift of food and the gift of your own body. You will not win the battle if I go easy on you and say, "Oh, go ahead and stuff in those French fries, that double cheeseburger, that donut, that giant convenience-store soda. But just eat that stuff a few times per week."

You know that strategy will never work. You will remain hooked, addicted to those foods and drinks forever. You have to break that cycle completely, and that means a radical change of diet.

Eating Healthy at Home

What if my mom won't cooperate, you ask. What if she won't buy any healthy foods and, no matter what I say, and insists on bringing home tons of snack food and calorie-packed desserts? Well, if she won't listen to your request for healthier eating, she's very, very unusual. And she's responsible for her behavior. However, you're probably one of the 95 percent of kids whose mother will be thrilled that you want to eat healthier.

Please don't go into an eternal state of mourning because you think you'll never be able to eat delicious foods again. There are hundreds of cookbooks packed with recipes that are good for you and still taste terrific. Plan to reward yourself once or twice a week with a low-sugar or natural-sugar dessert.

Below are some cookbooks with unbelievably cool recipes that you'll love. Show the titles to your mom. She can order them off any Internet bookstore such as Barnes & Noble, Amazon, Borders, Books-a-Million, etc. These sites also offer used copies of the books at reduced prices. You might even find these in thrift stores or used bookshops.

- *Betty Crocker's Eat and Lose Weight*
- *Weight Watchers New Complete Cookbook*
- *Weight Watchers All-Time Favorites: Over 200 Best-ever Recipes from the Weight Watchers Test Kitchens*
- *Suzanne Somer's Eat Great; Lose Weight*
- *Suzanne Somer's Get Skinny on Fabulous Food*
- *McDougall Quick and Easy Cookbook: Over 300 Delicious, Low-fat Recipes you can Prepare in 15 Minutes or Less,* by John and Mary McDougall
- *New Dieter's Cookbook* (Better Homes and Gardens)
- *Biggest Loser Cookbook: More than 125 Healthy, Delicious Recipes Adapted from NBC's Hit Show,* by Devin Alexander, Karen Kaplan
- *Sweet! From Agave to Turbinado: Home Baking with Every Kind of Natural Sugar and Sweetener,* by Manu Niall

Let me clarify something: I am not telling you to go on a particular diet. There are hundreds of diet plans out there. I've tried and failed so on many of them that I think it's silly for me to recommend yet another weird diet. What I'm encouraging and challenging you to do is just start eating healthy food. Bug your mom until she starts making healthier meals with fresh vegetables and fruits, whole grains, cereals and breads, lean meats, low sugar/low fat desserts—just an overall healthy diet every day.

I'm also not telling you that if you ever touch sugar again you'll blimp out! Skinny people can be just as unhealthy as someone who battles a weight problem. What we're trying to learn to do is eat healthier. As you know, one of my biggest battles happened to be with sugar. Working sugar out of my eating plan took time. If you're serious about losing weight, you may need to look at sugar as an addiction. Call it your "sweet trap." Educate yourself, watch your eating habits, recognize your traps, and then begin training yourself to overcome them one at a time. I like to call this retraining the mind. You are the one in control of your eating, not the sugar, the fat, the calories, or any other obstacle. Remember, you have been feeding your body certain foods for a very long time and bad habits are hard to break. But they can be broken!

Out on the Town

You might be thinking, "I may be able to begin controlling what I eat at home, but what about when I eat out?" Fabulous question. Making healthy food choices at fast food places, restaurants, and friends' homes is a special concern. First of all, try not to eat out too often. If you do, it could make losing weight a lot more challenging.

When you do eat out, it's really tough to control calories and fat, especially at fast food joints. But many of them now offer fresh fruit, salads, unbattered, non-deep fried meats, lite wraps instead of big sandwiches, lite entrees, etc. In restaurants, go for vegetable or fruit salads or the salad bar. Order broiled seafood instead of fried; order grilled chicken instead of those fatty ribs, sauce-slathered entrees, or prime rib. For side dishes, ask if you can have a double portion of the veggie of the day, steamed, instead of that monster baked potato or the French fries. If you can't resist the baked potato, don't have it stacked with slabs of butter, sour cream, cheese, bacon bits, etc. Eat all your food so you'll be full, and then skip dessert.

If you eat in a friend's home, be polite. Try to eat at least a little of everything so nobody gets offended. But don't let the lady of the house keep talking you into piling on seconds and thirds.

Recognizing the Good Stuff

The kinds and amounts of food you eat determine how your body processes and responds to food. Let's take a look at my formerly favorite ingredient again: sugar. Obviously, it's important to keep your sugar intake as low as possible. Having a plan when you eat out can help you reach this goal. You need to understand the right amounts of carbohydrates (carbs) and fat you can allow for each meal. And let me add something that may surprise you: try not to skip meals, even if you only grab a piece of fruit for breakfast. When you skip a meal, it disrupts the way your body digests and uses food. Also, you will sometimes end up being starved at the next meal and scarf up way more food than you should.

I'm sure you've heard about the basic food groups. If possible, you should eat from each food group at every meal, if possible:

Basic Food Groups and Choices

- Grains: Bread and starches, including cereal, rice, and pasta: You may have six or more small servings per day. Eat brown rice and whole grains (wheat bread, oatmeal, whole grain breakfast cereals) instead of refined carbs (like white rice, potatoes with all the fixin's, white bread, sugary cereals, pasta)

- Fruits and vegetables: Select five to seven servings per day (apples, bananas, oranges, pears, berries, etc., and fresh veggies) Make small baggies of fruit for snacks and throw them into your backpack.
- Dairy: low-fat milk, yogurt, and cheese. This is so important for you as a teen. Drink 2% or fat-free milk. Yogurt is good for you, but be careful how much yogurt you eat because of the added sugar present in most yogurts. Choose good quality cheeses without much filler and go easy on the processed cheese or cheese slices.
- Protein: Meat, poultry, fish and eggs: Try not to eat more than three small servings of these per day (active boys may want to eat a slightly larger portions. Activity level is important. If you exercise very little, you'd best limit the size of your portions. I eat about a 4 oz. piece of meat, and right now, I'm not eating any beef. I occasionally eat chicken, turkey, or fish. This is just my personal choice. I also make sure I'm getting everything I need by including a good quality multi-vitamin daily. Lentils, beans, and nuts are an excellent source of low-calorie, low-fat, high-fiber protein and a great substitute for meat.
- Healthy fats: This is *so* important. Saturated fat/trans fat is your worst enemy, followed by polyunsaturated or hydrogenated fat. Check labels on food and try to cut these fats as much as possible out of your diet. Monounsaturated fats are okay. Eat things like nuts and avocados (I had to learn to like avocados). For cooking, use lite olive oil or canola oil. Piling certain salad dressings on a healthy salad can easily make it a high fat/high carb item. Look for lite salad dressings or, if you can learn to like it, do like I do and use fresh lemon juice on your salads.

Become a Food Label Reader

Every food sold in the grocery store is now required to include a label listing nutritional facts. It lists things like overall calories, grams of fat, carbohydrates, sugar, fiber, and protein.

Have you seen the Oreo Cakesters in your grocery aisle?

Here it is:

Nutrition Facts

Serving size: Two Cakesters

Calories: 260 Calories from fat: 100

Saturated fat: 3 grams

Trans fat: 0g (Yeah!)
Polyunsaturated fat: 25g
Monounsaturated fat: 6g
(Four different types of fat that total 34g of fat).
Carbohydrates: 36g
Protein: 2 g
Dietary fiber: 1g
Sugars: 26g

Ingredients: (the first five ingredients are: Sugar, Enriched unbleached and bleached flour, canola oil and or Palm oil and/or Palm kernel oil, skim milk, fructose. (By the way, do you know that ingredients are listed in the order of amount—starting with the most.)

Following the first five ingredients we have: High fructose corn syrup Chocolate, Cornstarch, Egg whites, Salt, Corn syrup, Flavorings, Eggs, Soy lecithin, Corn flour, Preservatives and chemicals to preserve freshness

So you have two snack cakes that weigh 6 oz. each. A total of 12 oz. 130 calories each, and absolutely no nutrition. Approximately 65 calories a bite!

The package is attractive, inviting, conveniently packaged—very appealing. The cost to our health: zero nutritional value with a ton of carbs and sugar.

Now let's look at an example of a healthy snack
Blue Diamond Almonds
Ingredients: whole natural almonds
1 oz. package (snack bags) 1 serving (approximately 25 nuts)
Calories: 160
Total fat: 14 grams
Saturated fat: 1g
Trans fat: 0g
Potassium: 210mg
Total carbs: 6g
Dietary fiber: 3g
Sugar: 1g
Protein: 6g

This is an excellent snack for between meals, while you prepare your meal, or slivered and sprinkled on top of your vegetable. It's healthy and it will aid you in maintaining a level feeling of being full and satisfied. Lots of Leptin.

Now let's look at an easy-to-fix, healthy meal – Chicken Vegetable Stir Fry.

Birdseye, stir fry vegetables (frozen pepper stir fry)
Ingredients: green, red, and yellow bell peppers, onions
Calories 25 per serving (1 serving equals 1 cup)
5 servings in package
Total calories: 125
Total fat: 0
Total carbs: 5g
Dietary fiber: 1g
Sugars: 3g

Tyson Chicken Breast (frozen)
Ingredients: boneless, skinless chicken breast
Calories 100 (per 3oz serving) 2-4 servings per package
Total fat: 1.5g
Trans fat: 0g
Polyunsaturated fat: 1g
Monounsaturated fat: 1g
Cholesterol: 55mg
Total carbs: 3g
Dietary fiber: 0g
Sugars: 1g

Chop up the chicken into bite-size pieces. Measure 1 T. of canola or virgin olive oil, heat in pan. Add stir-fry vegetables and cook on fairly high heat, 3-5 minutes. I add my chicken at the same time. I sometimes add extra onion and seasonings to my liking.

While you're cooking, munch on some of those almonds. These really help curb your appetite. Eat them as a snack about 15-20 minutes before meals. This really works.

Within minutes, you will have a healthy, delicious meal, including the almonds, with a total of 485 calories. You can eat the entire meal or divide it into two servings, using the second serving as one of your snacks. I like to stuff this into a pita pocket.

Some of you are wrinkling your noses. I don't like this stuff, yuk! It takes too much time to cook, and the best excuse: my family won't eat it. I said the same things.

Why don't we want to eat a meal like this? It's healthy, low in calories, sugar free, the right kind of fat. It will actually fill you up and give you that level feeling of satisfaction for a very long time.

So why do the majority of us turn up our noses? Because our bodies are so used to the wrong foods. It will take a little time to begin really liking healthier ones. We also have learned to dislike certain foods, perhaps since childhood, when our parents didn't insist that we eat foods we weren't used to. Believe me, there are many foods you will learn to love if you just start slow and easy. Eat small portions of foods you're not sure you like until you begin developing a taste for them.

To Summarize the Fit for Life plan:

1. Change what you eat.
2. Cut down your food portion size and eat healthy snacks.
3. Regain control and exercise your authority.
4. Put your faith into action.
5. Start exercising regularly. Walking is the easiest and least expensive form of exercise. Start with a short distance and go from there.
6. Search for a support person or group, or start one of your own within your school or church family.
7. God has given us many tools and the best one of all is His Word. Read it daily.

Good luck. There is only one way for you—SUCCESS! When you fall, get right back up, brush off the dust, and get back in the saddle.

And I am sure that God, who began the good work within you, will continue his work until it is finally finished on that day when Christ Jesus comes back again.

--- Philippians 1:6

Final Exam

The purpose of this course was not to fill your head with facts, but to offer you a Bible-based plan for healthy living. That being the case, this final exam will be open-book. Some of the questions pertain to your current personal health journey. It will be up to you to evaluate your progress and "grade yourself" accordingly.

1. Obesity or being way out of shape is mostly just an adult problem in the United States.
   _________True _________ False

2. In 2 Corinthians 7:1 we are challenged to cleanse ourselves from anything that ____________ our body or spirit.

3. What does Wyndy, the author, mean when she talks about the "Trap" that she discovered? ____
   ____
   ____

4. When Eve took a bite of the fruit in the Garden, she was really taking the first human bite of _________.

5. In what two main areas does Satan use to trap us into sinning? The ____________ and the ____.

6. The World is the evil society around us and the Flesh is our own tendency to make wrong decisions against what God wants. True _________ False _________.

7. Satan knows that if he can control your body, he can also control your _________.

8. One sin we almost never hear anyone talk about is gluttony? What is gluttony?
 ____

9. A verse that will help us when we're tempted to sin is James 4:7: "So humble yourselves before God, ____________ the devil, and he will ____________ from you."

10. When God told Adam and Eve not to eat of one particular fruit in the Garden of Eden, it was to protect them from the knowledge of ____________ and ____________.

11. Today we humans know all about good and evil, and now there's a whole lot more than one food to tempt us. List at least five types of places around us daily that offer food:

12. Tempting food is everywhere. Can you list five events you attended in the past month in which tempting food was available?

13. What is Satan's responsibility as the 'head chef' of unhealthy eating?

14. You may be tempted to think that it's a little crazy to imagine that Satan cares about the kinds and amounts of food we eat. But if he can cause us to ruin our bodies and our health, how would this help his kingdom and hurt God's kingdom?

15. In your own words, tell the story of Daniel and his quest for a healthy diet in Babylon:

16. What happened to the manna of the Israelites when they tried to hoard it so they could stuff themselves?

17. List some of the foods God promised to give the Israelites in the Promised Land:

18. Were the foods healthy or unhealthy? ______________________________

19. We already know Satan tries to ruin our souls. List three strategies Satan uses to destroy our bodies:

20. What are three paths through which Satan tries to abuse us emotionally?

21. Which one of the choices below does Satan ***not*** try to steal from us?

    a. Our favorite fried foods   b. Our self-control

    c. Our joy   d. Our authority

22. If your will power and authority does not belong to you by God's power, who does it belong to?

23. Does Satan destroy people instantly or gradually? ______________________

24. How can foods destroy us gradually? ______________________________

25. What part of us does Satan infiltrate to influence us? ____________________

26. The hypothalamus is that part of the brain in which our appetite for drugs is regulated. True __________ False __________

27. ____________ is a chemical that shuts off your hunger and stimulates you to burn more calories.

28. ____________ is a chemical that is released through your hormones when your stomach is empty and it makes you want to eat.

29. We want to keep our Leptin levels high and our Ghrelin levels non-functioning. True ____________ False ____________

30. The Bible teaches that you, as a Christian, are a temple of God. What does that mean?

31. What does it mean if we say that a person is disciplined?

32. How can a person become more disciplined?

33. Summarize the 3 steps for becoming disciplined and taking authority over your eating habits.

    a.

    b.

    c.

34. Explain how the movie Karate Kid illustrates the importance of personal discipline.

35. What does the author mean by saying that living wisely can result in life and radiant health?

36. List four things you can do or say to resist the temptations of unhealthy foods pressed on you by friends and family.

    a.

    b.

    c.

    d.

37. Read Romans 14:10. Remember, it is not your duty to start telling your parents, friends, brothers or sisters that they have to eat exactly the same foods you've decided to eat. Don't get mad and condemn them. They must make their own decisions about food and it's between them and God.

    Write about how the people in your life are reacting to your new way of eating:

38. Just as Jesus' Father gave Him authority on earth, Jesus has also given us, as Christians, His authority or power. When we claim the power of Jesus Christ, Satan is ____________________ against us.

39. Satan can only take as much power over us as we let him.
    True ____________ False ____________.

40. Battles are won and lost in our ____________.

41. How is Satan like a lion in our lives?

42. How does putting on the armor of God help you win the battle over eating too much and eating the wrong foods?

43. These three gates must be checked every day: the food you ____________, the food you ________________________________, and the food you ____________.

44. We've read about this since the course started. What should be done immediately if we sin? ____

45. Repentance isn't just being sorry. It is being sorry enough to ____________. Because of what Jesus did for us on the cross, sin's power over us is ____________.

46. What are three rules we must follow to avoid sin?
    a. Do not let sin ____________ the way you live.
    b. Do not give in to its ________________________________.
    c. Do not let any part of your ____________ become a tool of ________________ to be used for sinning.

47. Whatever you choose to obey becomes your ________________________.

48. In the book of James, we're warned against the destructive words our tongues can say about others and to others. But our tongue also includes our sense of ____________. When foods taste good, we're tempted to eat them, not just occasionally, but all the time.

49. List five ways you can tame your tongue in regard to food:
    a.
    b.
    c.
    d.
    e.

50. The main point of this course is that food is bad and eating is sinful. True __________ False __________

51. List five suggestions given to help you control the foods you eat when you eat out:
    a.
    b.
    c.
    d.
    e.

52. Name the 5 basic food groups: ____________ ____________

    ____________ ____________ ____________

    From which food group do you eat the most? ____________
    The least? ____________

53. What one change can you make today that would result in your eating a more balanced diet? ____________

54. Choose three items from your kitchen that you eat frequently. Examine the nutrition facts: calories, grams of saturated fat and grams of monounsaturated fats, grams of protein, fiber, sugar and carbs. Create totals of approximately how many calories, fat grams, and carb/sugar grams you would be eating if you consumed one serving of all three in a meal.

55. The Fit for Life Summary: (fill in the blanks)
    a. Change what you ____________.
    b. Cut down your food ____________ size and eat ____________ snacks.
    c. Regain control and exercise your ____________.
    d. Put your ____________ into action.
    e. Start ____________ regularly. Walking is the easiest and least expensive form of this. Start with a short distance and go from there.
    f. Search for a ____________ person or group, or start one of your own within your school or church family.
    g. God has given us many tools and the best one of all is ____________. Read it daily.

56. Place a check mark beside the excuses you've made for not eating right:
   a. _________I'm overweight because obesity runs in my family.
   b. _________I can't help being overweight; it's just a chemical imbalance in my body.
   c. _________I'm unhealthy because my parents are unhealthy. There's nothing I can do about it.
   d. _________I'm naturally a large-boned person. I need a lot of food to fill my body.
   f. _________I've tried diets and they just don't work for me.

57. When a hunter sets a trap, he baits it with something to entice the prey for the purpose of being caught. When you think of a trap for animals, what comes to mind as the type of object often used as bait? ______________________________

58. The Devil's Trap (his plan to deceive) also involves bait.
   a. What kinds of food does he usually bait your trap with? ________________
   ____
   b. Where does he put his traps in order to catch you? ________________
   ____

59. Place a check mark next to the things you have done so far to begin winning the battle over food.
   a. _________I've recognized my unhealthy habits as sin and I have admitted this to God and repented.
   b. _________I've decided to change my eating habits
   c. _________My mom and I have discussed the kinds of foods that are more healthy and have agreed to begin reading food labels to buy healthier foods with less fat and less calories.
   d. _________I've found a partner with whom I can be accountable so we can help each other become healthier (your mom, sister, friend, etc. If you haven't found anyone yet, that's okay.)
   e. _________I have changed my between-meal snacks to healthier ones.
   f. _________I am beginning to keep a daily food journal about what I eat, how I can eat better, and how things are going to reach my goals of losing weight and getting in shape.

g. _________ I have decided on the kind of exercise that is best for me and is practical to be able to do every day. That kind is: _________

h. _________ I have begun my exercise program (walking a mile, doing calisthenics, jogging, doing aerobics, playing tennis or some other sport, etc.) I exercise for _________ minutes _________ times per week.

i. _________ I have lost at least one pound of body weight since beginning this course.

j. _________ I have lost at least five pounds of body weight since beginning this course.

60. Explain your understanding of the author's revelation of The Trap, The Plague, and the Dwelling. (Essay question)

References

Oz, Mehmet and M. Roizen. *You: On a Diet; The Owner's Manual for Waist Management.* New York: Free Press, 2006.

Student Notebook Webster's Dictionary. New York: HarperCollins Publishers, Inc., 2004.

Your Personal Journal

Teacher's Supplement for Fit for Life Curriculum

There is a dangerous epidemic in our nation. It is manifesting itself in children and teens who are overweight, sedentary, out-of-shape, or downright obese. Some are already experiencing early signs of diabetes, high cholesterol, depression, and high blood pressure. Even scarier, an overweight kid may eventually become one of the 300,000 Americans who die each year due to medical complications caused by obesity.

Wyndy Buckner struggled for many years, until she discovered a plan that enabled her to lose 75 lbs. This course for teens teaches the spiritual as well as the dietary principles that enabled her to reclaim her life and health. Every Christian teen who struggles with weight issues, or any teen desiring to live a healthy lifestyle, should consider taking this inspiring and practical course.

Fit for Life will work well as an elective or as a supplement to health, nutrition, science, and/or Bible curricula.

Students can work independently with minimal instruction as the workbook is interactive and encourages self-discovery through journaling and inductive Bible study. Teachers may choose to check progress by assigning a certain number of pages or chapter per week, by checking journal entries, or by pop quizzes selected from the final exam questions. A periodic class discussion about the material might also help students to open up about their health issues and concerns.

Other options for teachers to expand the lessons might include assignments to plan and prepare healthy meals at home; field trips to the grocery store/evaluating food labels; a health-walk activity; swimming; a visit to a local gym, etc.

Students are free to use any Bible version of their choice. The author predominantly uses the New Living Translation.

Students are also free to use any dictionary available to them. Both a Bible and a dictionary are necessary for the work in this course. A journal is recommended.

Answer Key to Final Exam

1. Obesity or being way out of shape is mostly just an adult problem in the United States. **False**

2. In 2 Corinthians 7:1 we are challenged to cleanse ourselves from anything that **defiles** our body or spirit.

3. What does Wyndy, the author, mean when she talks about the "Trap" that she discovered? **The Traps are ways we are tempted to abuse our bodies by avoiding healthy foods and eating unhealthy ones.**

4. Our lesson shows how, when Eve took a bite of the fruit in the Garden, she was really taking the first human bite of **sin**.

5. What two areas does Satan use to trap us into sinning? The **World** and the **Flesh**

6. The World is the evil society around us and the Flesh is our own tendency to make wrong decisions against what God wants. **True**

7. Satan knows that if he can control your body, he can also control your **thoughts.**

8. One sin we almost never hear anyone talk about is gluttony. What is gluttony? **Gluttony is overeating or gorging oneself on more food and drink that we should.**

9. One verse that will help us when we're tempted to sin is James 4:7: "So humble yourselves before God, **resist** the devil, and he will flee from you."

10. When God told Adam and Eve not to eat of one particular fruit in the Garden of Eden, it was to protect them from the knowledge of **good and evil.**

11. Today we humans know all about good and evil, and now there's a whole lot more than one food to tempt us. List at least five types of places around us daily that offer food: (note, students may list others at their discretion)
fast food joints
restaurants
grocery stores
malls
donut shops

12. Can you list five events you attended in the past month in which food was available?
Answers will vary

13. What is Satan's responsibility as the 'head chef' of unhealthy eating?
To destroy our bodies so he can also damage us spiritually and emotionally

14. You may be tempted to think that it's a little crazy to think that Satan cares about the kinds and amounts of food we eat. But if he can cause us to ruin our bodies and our health, how would this help his kingdom and hurt God's kingdom?
We would be lazier, slower, less efficient, out of shape—poor examples of how much better life can be with Christ.

15. In your own words, tell the story of Daniel and his quest for a healthy diet in Babylon:
Here is one version: As a captured Jew in Babylon, Daniel asked the head honcho if he could test him and his friends for a period of time with a healthy diet. When the period of time ended, they looked much healthier than those who ate the king's rich, fatty foods.

16. What happened to the manna of the Israelites when they tried to hoard it so they could stuff themselves? **It spoiled and smelled rotten**

17. List some of the foods God promised to give the Israelites in the Promised Land:
    Grains
    Fruit: such as grapes, wine etc.
    Vegetables: such as olives, etc.
    Meat: such as beef and goat meat
    Dairy: such as cow's milk, goat's milk, etc.

18. Were the foods healthy or unhealthy? **Healthy**

19. We know Satan tries to ruin our souls. List a few of the strategies Satan uses to destroy our bodies: **Disease, eating disorders, obesity, addictions, high blood pressure, etc.**

20. What are three paths through which Satan tries to abuse us emotionally?
    Our self-worth, our joy, and our self-control.

21. Which of the choices below does Satan *not* try to steal from us?
    a. Our favorite fried foods b. Our self-control
    c. Our joy d. Our authority

22. If your will power and authority does not belong to you by God's power, to whom does it belong? **Satan**

23. Does Satan destroy people instantly or gradually? **Both, but it is usually very gradual throughout a lifetime.**

24. How can unhealthy foods destroy us gradually? **Through such things as heart disease, organ dysfunction, high blood pressure, diabetes**

25. What part of us does Satan infiltrate to influence us? **Our mind**

26. The hypothalamus is that part of the brain in which our appetite for drugs is regulated. **True.**

27. **Leptin** shuts off your hunger and stimulates you to burn more calories.

28. **Ghrelin** is a chemical that is released through your hormones when your stomach is empty and it makes you want to eat.

29. We want to keep our Leptin levels high and our Ghrelin levels non-functioning. **True**

30. The Bible teaches that you, as a Christian, are a temple of God. What does that mean exactly? **God's Spirit lives inside of us.**

31. What does it mean if I say that a person is 'disciplined'?
It means he or she has a lot of will power

32. How can a person become more disciplined?
Saying no to yourself more and more when needed, really meaning it, and sticking to it

33. Summarize the three steps for being disciplined and taking authority over your eating habits.
    a. **Make a "recipe" card and write on it several Scriptures that apply to your problem.**
    b. **Set a few eating goals that you want to achieve.**
    c. **Decide how you're going to avoid the unhealthy foods and eat healthy ones.**

34. Explain how the movie, Karate Kid, illustrates the importance of personal discipline.
Danny learns that when Mr. Miyagi made him do really tough chores, he was actually making him stronger, more disciplined, and better able to face challenges in life.

35. What does the author mean by saying that living wisely can result in life and radiant health? **Life is the active principle of existence.**
Radiant health is a sound, well-conditioned body.

36. List four things you can do so these temptations won't cause you to do what you don't want to do:
   a. **Plan your strategy.**
   b. **Decide daily what you will eat.**
   c. **Be prepared in advance.**
   d. **Don't stray from your plan.**

37. Read Romans 14:10. Remember, it is not your duty to start telling your parents, friends, brothers or sisters that they have to eat exactly the same foods you've decided to eat. Don't get mad and condemn them. They must make their own decisions about food and it's between them and God.
   Write about how the people in your life are reacting to your new way of eating:
   Answers will vary.

38. Just as Jesus' Father gave Him authority on earth, Jesus has also given us, as Christians, His authority or power. When we claim the power of Jesus Christ, Satan is **powerless** against us.

39. Satan can only take as much power over us as we let him. **True**

40. Battles are won and lost in our **heart** or **mind**.

41. How is Satan like a lion in our lives? **He searches for the young, the weak, or the sickly. He strikes quickly and brutally.**

42. How does putting on the armor of God help you win the battle over eating too much and eating the wrong foods?
   Answers will vary. For example, the Shield of Faith can stop Satan's temptations. The Sword of the Spirit (the Word) can rebuke the Traps of the Enemy. The Helmet of Salvation can protect (guard) our minds.

43. These three gates must be checked every day: the food you **see,** the food you **hear about**, and the food you **eat.**

44. We've read about this since the course started. What should be done immediately if we sin? **Repent from it, and start over.**

45. Repentance isn't just being sorry. It is being sorry enough to **change.** Because of what Jesus did for us on the Cross sins power over us is **broken.**

46. What are three rules we must follow to avoid sin?
    a. **Do not let sin control the way you live.**
    b. **Do not give in to its lustful desire.**
    c. **Do not let any part of your body become a tool of wickedness to be used for sinning.**

47. Whatever you choose to obey becomes your **master**.

48. In the book of James, we're warned against the destructive words our tongues can say about others and to others. But our tongue also includes our sense of **taste.** When foods taste good, we're tempted to eat them, not just occasionally, but all the time.

49. List five ways we can tame our tongue in regard to food. Whatever things are:
    a. Healthy
    b. Good for you
    c. Small in portion
    d. Under the authority of God's Word
    e. Controlled

50. The main point of this course is that food is bad and eating is sinful. **False**

51. List five suggestions given to help you control the foods you eat when you eat out:
    a. Order fresh fruit or a salad
    b. Order unbattered, non-deep fried foods
    c. Eat broiled or baked seafood instead of fried
    d. Eat lite wraps instead of big sandwiches
    e. Ask for a double portion of the veggies instead of potato or rice

52. Name the 5 basic food groups. **Grains, Fruits/Vegetables, Dairy, Proteins, Fats.** From which food group do you eat the most? **Answers will vary.** From which group do you eat the least? **Answers will vary.**

53. What one change can you make today that would result in your eating a more balanced diet? ____

54. Choose three items from your kitchen that you eat frequently. Examine the nutrition facts: calories, grams of saturated fat and grams of monounsaturated fats, grams of protein, fiber, sugar and carbs. Create totals of approximately how many calories, fat grams, and carb/sugar grams you would be eating if you consumed one serving of all three in a meal.

55. The Fit for Life Summary. Fill in the blanks

    1. Change what you **eat.**
    2. Cut down your food **portion size** and eat **healthy** snacks.
    3. Regain control and exercise your **authority.**
    4. Put your **faith** into action.
    5. Start **exercising** regularly. Walking is the easiest and least expensive form of this. Start with a short distance and go from there.
    6. Search for a **support** person or group, or start one of your own within your school or church family.
    7. God has given us many tools and the best one of all is **His Word**. Read it daily.

    Personal Evaluation Section:

56. Place a check mark beside the excuses you've made for not eating right:

    a. ______ I'm overweight because obesity runs in my family. My relatives are overweight.
    b. ______ I can't help being overweight; it's just a chemical imbalance in my body.
    c. ______ I'm unhealthy because my parents are unhealthy. There's nothing we can do about it.
    d. ______ I'm naturally a large-boned person. I need a lot of food to fill my body.
    e. ______ I've tried diets and they just don't work for me.

    Responses will vary from person to person.

57. When a hunter sets a trap, he first baits it with something to entice the prey. When you think of a trap for animals, what comes to mind as the type of object often used as bait? **Usually it's some type of food.**

58. The Devil's Trap (his plan to deceive) also often includes food.

c. What kinds of food does he usually bait your trap with?

Answers will vary.

d. Where does he put his traps in order to catch you?

Answers will vary.

59. Place a check mark next to the things you have done so far to begin winning the battle over food.

(Students will mark this according to their progress so far.)

a. ______ I've recognized my unhealthy habits as sin and I have admitted this to God and repented.

b. ______ I've decided to change my eating habits and having healthier meals.

c. ______ My mom and I have discussed the kinds of foods that are more healthy and have agreed to begin reading food labels to buy healthier foods with less fat and less calories.

d. ______ I've found a partner with whom I can be accountable so we can help each other become healthier (your mom, sister, friend, etc. If you haven't found anyone, that's OK.)

e. ______ I have changed my between-meal snacks to healthier ones.

f. ______ I am beginning to keep a daily food journal about what I eat, how I can eat better, and how things are going to reach my goals of losing weight and getting in shape.

g. ______ I have decided on the kind of exercise that is best for me and is practical to be able to do every day.

h. ______ I have begun my exercise program (walking a mile, doing calisthenics, jogging, doing aerobics, playing tennis or some other sport, etc.)

i. ______ I have lost at least one pound of body weight.

j. ______ I have lost at least five pounds of body weight.

60. Explain your understanding of the author's revelation of The Trap, The Plague, and the Dwelling.

Answers will vary.